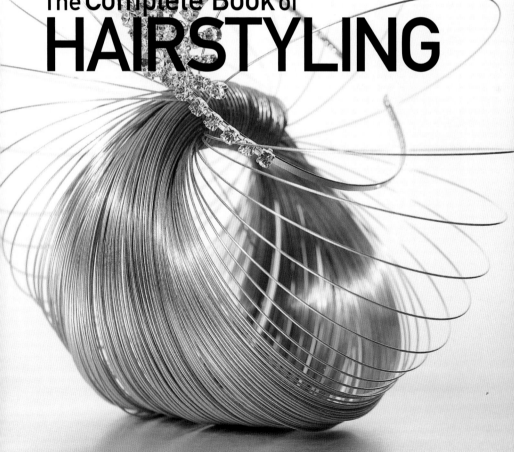

The Complete Book of
HAIRSTYLING

THIS IS A CARLTON BOOK

Text (except City Hair pages 12, 32, 56, 80 and Big Date Hair), design, illustrations
and photography copyright © 2001 Carlton Books Limited
Text City Hair pages 12, 32, 56, 80 and Big Date Hair copyright © 2001 Karen Wheeler
Original idea and concept copyright © 2001 Charles Worthington Limited

This edition published by Carlton Books Limited 2011
20 Mortimer Street
London W1T 3JW

10 9 8 7 6 5 4 3 2 1

A CIP catalogue record for this book is available from the British Library

ISBN 978-1-84732-718-5

The author, licensor and publisher have made every effort to ensure that all information is correct and
up to date at the time of publication. Neither the author, licensor or publisher can accept responsibility
for any accident, injury or damage that results from using the ideas, information or advice offered.

The application and quality of hair products and treatments, herbal preparations and essential oils
is beyond the control of the above parties, who cannot be held responsible for any problems resulting
from their use. Always follow the manufacturer's instructions and if in doubt seek further advice.

Do not use herbal preparations or essential oils without prior consultation with a qualified practitioner or
medical doctor if you are pregnant, taking any form of medication or if you suffer from oversensitive skin.
Half-doses of essential oils should always be used for children and the elderly.

No resemblance is intended to any person, living or dead, in the fiction element of this book.
The events and the characters who take part in them have no relation to actual events or living people.

Text: Carmel Allen (City Hair), Karen Wheeler (Big Date Hair),
Emma Craven (Holiday Hair) and Lisa Helmanis (Big Day Hair)
Photographer (model): Hugh Arnold
Photographer (still life): Patrice de Villiers
Illustrator: Jason Brooks
Stylists: Sophie Kenningham and Rachel Davis
Make-up: Chase Aston and Maggie Hunt
Editorial Manager: Venetia Penfold
Art Director: Penny Stock
Senior Art Editor: Barbara Zuñiga
Project Editor: Zia Mattocks
Production: Kate Pimm

Printed and bound in China

The Complete Book of

HAIRSTYLING

Charles Worthington

CARLTON
BOOKS

contents

foreword

I defy anyone to underestimate the power of hair and its ability to transform the way you look and feel! Your hair is your most important fashion accessory and the first thing that people notice about you. It speaks volumes about your personality, lifestyle, look and, most of all, what sort of mood you're in: casual and laid-back, minimal and understated, glamorous and sexy, sleek and neat or wild and va-va-voom. What's important to me, as a hairdresser who has witnessed and enjoyed the buzz that people get from a great cut or a new style, is to make fabulous hair accessible to everyone every day of the year. The aim is to make sure you can enjoy hair that is in peak condition and fulfilling its maximum potential whether you're at home, away on holiday, preparing for a change of image or planning your wedding. Most of all, though, I think hair should be fun – it should be about enjoying your individuality and finding a hairstyle that suits you and your lifestyle.

polly

jaz

Polly is a City career babe – traditional, yes, but she's got a twist. Her double first in maths means she can tot up her buying splurges as fast as the computers at Visa. She always looks immaculate and only her closest friends know that her sleek blonde hair is the result of painstaking styling to iron out its natural wave. Polly's money-mad boyfriend Harry is inclined to insensitivity and it's beginning to get her down. She needs something – or someone – to inject a bit of excitement into her life. Everyone thinks she's as straight as her hair, but she's about to show them a new side to her character.

Jaz (short for Jasmine) is your regular club bunnie. She loves all things hip, cool and girlie. Her earliest memory is of dressing up in the contents of her mother's overstuffed wardrobe – and clothes are still her greatest passion. She can't remember the last time she took off her make-up before going to bed but, with her long, thick, glossy black hair, she always looks stunning nevertheless. Always the party girl, Jaz will try anything once and dreams of landing herself a high-glamour job in fashion. She's not fussy, as long as it fuels her passion for fashion, fun and trying out new hairstyles.

kate

laura

Kate looks like a pre-Raphaelite painting: unruly curly titian hair, milky complexion and rosy cheeks. She works as a personal assistant to the marketing director of Crunch Biscuits – not a good career choice when you have a sweet tooth and are prone to overindulgence. Kate is a hopeless romantic with an insatiable crush on her boss. But spending hours daydreaming of weekends away with him in exotic destinations isn't getting her anywhere. It's time to make some changes, and it's not just her looks and love life that are in need of a revamp, her career needs something of a kick-start, too.

Laura is a tomboy: lean and androgynous with a short crop. Her uniform is urban cool – more combats and trainers than pencil skirts and kitten heels. She wouldn't be seen dead in anything glittery. Laura loves to work out but is fiercely competitive and intimidates most of her fellow gym-goers. A struggling TV researcher who wants to make gritty documentaries and dreams of winning a BAFTA, Laura's recognized the benefits of networking. She's also trying to attract the attention of a certain assistant producer and decides that a redefined image – still tomboy but with a feminine twist – just might be the answer.

city hair

Discover the **perfect** haircare routine to suit your particular **needs**, cuts to enhance your face shape, colours to **complement** your **skin tone** and just-left-the-salon **styling** techniques to help you achieve and **maintain** salon-style hair every day of the week. City Hair **answers** your everyday hair needs, whether it's **redefining** your **image** to help you get **ahead** at work, coping with 'stressed' **hair** or getting caught out with a **last-minute** after-work **party** invitation.

hair basics

home, sweet home

'**Oh, Polly,' moaned Kate,** tossing back her unruly red curls and flinging herself down perilously on Polly's new cream sofa, glass of red wine in hand. 'I can't believe you've agreed to let Chrissie come and stay for a month – what a nightmare.' Polly did indeed know that Chrissie could be high-maintenance (to say the least), but then so, too, could Kate. She grimaced as a drop of wine from Kate's glass splashed onto her candy-striped pyjamas, but at least it didn't hit the sofa.

With the help of her parents (rich) and her first city bonus, Perfect Polly – as the others called her in their more green-eyed moments – had bought a four-bedroom house in Shepherd's Bush, chosen largely for its proximity to fashionable, but much more expensive, Notting Hill. Polly had proceeded to install her BFs: Laura, her best friend from Manchester University and her two oldest friends from school in Southampton, fashion-mad Jaz and, of course, Kate. Playing the part of landlady to what seemed like a bunch of teenagers at times was enough to make Polly's cool blonde locks curl at the ends even more than they were prone to do naturally.

'Oh, come on, Kate. Don't you remember what fun Chrissie was at school?' said Jaz, who was looking forward to having someone to swap the latest make-up tips with. Jaz was also eager to update her long curtain of thick black hair inherited from her Indian mother, and Chrissie, a beauty therapist on Virtual Airlines, would be able to fill her in on all the latest looks in New York.

'She'll hog the bathroom and leave her make-up and clothes all over the place,' said Kate grumpily. 'And she'll steal everyone's boyfriend.'
'Polly's the only one among us who's got a boyfriend,' said Laura, looking up from her book on the mating habits of otters. Laura, a TV researcher on a wildlife programme, could always be relied upon to be blunt (rather like her boyish crop). But having never actually met the infamous Chrissie, she had no strong views on her imminent arrival. Instead, she asked, 'Why is she coming to stay, Pol? I thought she was based in New York now.'
'Something to do with a record producer she met on one of her transatlantic flights,' said Polly. 'Apparently he's promised to get her an audition with a new girl band.'
'Oh, for God's sake,' said Kate, who, if the truth be told, was more than a little jealous of Chrissie's thin thighs and exciting life. Her own thighs were not so svelte (thanks to her sweet tooth), while her job as a PA at Crunch Biscuits couldn't be more boring.

Polly, meanwhile, was looking forward to a little distraction (her boyfriend Harry certainly wasn't providing it) and Chrissie was bound to liven things up at 23 Havana Road ...

head start

Nothing reflects inner health, vitality and wellbeing quite like a clear complexion, sparkling eyes and – your crowning glory – glossy hair. Beauty comes from within, and if you have an unhealthy diet and lifestyle, your hair – like your skin – will suffer. Tiredness and stress will also wreak havoc on your hair, so modern haircare must be holistic and take into account all aspects of your lifestyle. When you are tense, your scalp tightens and the blood capillaries contract, reducing the quantities of oxygen and nutrients that reach the hair follicles; the production of sweat increases, causing a greasy scalp; and, over prolonged periods of time, stress may even lead to hair loss. A good, relaxing scalp massage can help maintain a healthy head of hair, relieving tension and increasing blood flow, which will, in turn, nourish the root and hair follicle (see page 26 for how to do it).

Clean, shiny hair is a joy to have and head-turning to watch. Yet how often have we been told that our hair is dead, that it is just a build-up of deceased protein cells, strands of keratin which feel no pain when they're cut? This much is true. But hair is also organic in the same way as leather or wood is organic. Just think of how a favourite pair of shoes responds to a good polish, or how a wooden surface shines after a little elbow grease and beeswax. Nourish and condition them and they will shine, 'breathe' and last for years. With the same love and attention, so will your hair. Taking care of your locks is a threefold affair: providing nourishment, treating it with care and using the right products. The simple routines, tips and advice that follow will ensure that you have great salon-style hair every day.

food for thought
The bottom line is that you can't expect to have healthy hair if you eat unhealthily. Whatever products you put onto your tresses, the only real solution is a long-term one that comes from within – a varied diet full of essential vitamins, minerals and other nutrients. Your scalp – where the root and follicle are formed and where 'live'

hair grows and develops – forms part of your skin, the largest organ of the body but the last in the queue to receive nourishment from the food we eat (hence the number of skin creams that deliver vitamins and minerals topically). A poor diet means impoverished skin and scalp. If you know your diet is not balanced and you don't want to compromise the health of your hair, then supplement it with a vitamin B complex, antioxidants (including vitamins C, E and beta-carotene), gamma-linolenic acid (GLA), fish oil, linseed oil and the minerals selenium and zinc (see page 28 for more on this). Many pharmacies sell a good all-round hair and skin supplement.

gently does it
We wouldn't dream of tugging our favourite little black dress on over our head without undoing the zip, or putting our new silk undies in the tumble dryer for 30 minutes on a high heat setting. So why do we think nothing of committing similar crimes to our hair? Imagine your hair to be as precious as a cashmere twinset; treat it accordingly and you will reap the rewards. Brushwork is all-important: poor-quality brushes and combs will scratch the scalp and damage the hair shaft, so don't stint on these (see page 24). Hair is elastic to some extent, but too much pulling will overstretch and ultimately snap it, causing split ends.

no products, no style
Using the right products on your hair could make bad-hair days a thing of the past. The plethora on sale in any pharmacy, supermarket or salon makes choosing the ones appropriate for your hair type confusing. Slick advertising and packaging makes it even more difficult to get it right. Do you want to go herbal, organic, scientific, fruity or unscented? Will it make your hair bigger, softer, fuller, blonder or seal your split ends? The claims can often be overwhelming – and you just want your hair to look great. The first thing to do is to determine your hair type; once you've got that right, then you can think about the extras. Read on to find out how ...

hair types

Most people tend to wash their hair every day so they probably do not know exactly what hair type they have.

Your hair type is a combination of three factors:

1 The condition of your scalp – is it dry, oily or flaky?

2 The characteristics of your hair – is it fine, frizzy, coarse, curly, wavy, straight or colour-treated?

3 Your environment – do you live in the country or the city? Is your office air-conditioned? Is the climate hot and humid, wet and windy or dry and hot?

normal hair

If your hair is neither prone to oiliness or dryness, you are one of the lucky few to have normal hair. Look after it well with products that keep it clean, conditioned and protected from environmental damage.

combination hair

Five to six hours after washing, hair begins to show signs of oiliness around the root area and yet the ends of the hair remain dry. Oiliness can be caused by overuse of conditioners and styling products, as well as by humidity and pollution.

oily hair

The hair will look oily, dull and 'dirty' along the length of the hair shaft. If you suspect oily hair, make a parting and gently rub your forefinger along your scalp, then rub your thumb and forefinger together. If it feels slippery, you have an oily scalp and overactive sebum glands.

HAIR SNIP

TO CHECK WHICH HAIR TYPE YOU HAVE, WASH YOUR HAIR AS NORMAL AND LET IT DRY NATURALLY. THE NEXT MORNING, BEFORE WASHING YOUR HAIR AGAIN, CHECK FOR SIGNS OF DRYNESS OR OILINESS. YOUR HAIR TYPE WILL CHANGE IF IT CANNOT ADJUST NATURALLY TO CHANGES IN YOUR ENVIRONMENT. IT WILL ALSO PROBABLY CHANGE (BOTH SCALP AND HAIR SHAFT BECOMING DRIER) IF IT IS CHEMICALLY COLOURED OR PERMED.

dry hair

Dry hair will look dull, lifeless and parched; at its worst, it may look fuzzy and straw-like. If you suspect your scalp is dry, look at the white flakes on your shoulders before brushing them away. Small, powdery flakes are often the result of stress, too much alcohol and tiredness. If they are larger, translucent and moist, then it is a case of dandruff, due to overproduction of sebum in the hair follicles, rather than a dry scalp.

hair textures

curly hair

Often the cuticles (the overlapping keratin cells that form hair) do not lie flat on curly hair because of the curved nature of the shaft. This can lead to dull-looking hair and frizz. Overcome this with leave-in conditioners, serums and conditioning sprays.

afro hair

Afro hair is usually dry, brittle and fine. Hydrate the hair with conditioning preparations and massage the scalp gently to promote healthy growth and the production of sebum, the body's natural hair conditioner.

straight hair

The shaft of the hair is straight and, if the hair is in good condition and the cuticles are lying flat (the use of serum can encourage this), straight hair can look super-shiny. In less than ideal conditions, split ends and breakages may be noticeable.

coarse hair

This type of hair can look fuzzy and wiry after shampooing. Use a serum or leave-in conditioner to close and smooth the cuticle and do regular deep-conditioning treatments.

fine hair

Often this type of hair can look lank and lifeless soon after washing. Overconditioning will weigh the hair down, so only use it sparingly. Always use volumizing products especially formulated for fine hair.

chemically treated hair

Although colouring processes are more gentle than ever, some still change the make up of your hair permanently. Give coloured hair extra support by using rehydrating shampoos and conditioners that have been specifically designed for this hair type. Also, check that they contain sunscreen to protect your hair from damage caused by ultraviolet light and keep your colour looking fresh for longer.

dream routine

Compare your haircare regime to your skincare regime: face – cleanse, tone, moisturize and protect, apply make-up; hair – shampoo, condition and protect, style, finish. A shampoo will gently but effectively cleanse the hair shaft, while a conditioner will moisturize your hair like a good face cream moisturizes your skin. Appropriate styling and finishing products will protect it from heat and oxidation from ultraviolet light and pollution which create dangerous free radicals. There are more benefits to be had by following a four-step haircare regime – shampoo, condition, style, finish – than by relying only on a shampoo.

Few women skip a step in their skincare routine (are there still women who just use soap and water?) because modern products are designed to work together in synergy. The same is true of haircare products. Have you noticed how wonderful your hair looks when you have just been to the hairdressers and had the full treatment of shampoos, conditioners, styling products and finishing spray? Use them all regularly and your hair will become stronger, more flexible and resistant to damage. It's an accumulative effect.

shampoos

Beauty sceptics love to throw scorn on the relative merits of so-called designer shampoos. 'There's no difference between them and washing-up liquid,' is their collective cry. Well, they are wrong. Here's why. There is no denying that a bubble bath might share similar ingredients to a shampoo. But, as with humans whose bodies are made up of 90 per cent water and yet each one is unique, it is the other 10 per cent that makes all the difference. There are many special ingredients added to shampoos that can make hair look and behave as you would like, so experiment to find one that performs best for your hair type. Most modern shampoos are gentle enough to use every day and, in many cases, will actually improve the

condition of hair. It is not necessary to rub your hair like you might your clothes because the surfactant properties of the key ingredients in shampoos allow grime, dust, oil and dirt to lift away from the hair shaft, leaving your hair clean and porous for conditioning.

pH-balanced shampoos

Using a shampoo that is not pH-balanced could damage your hair, so make sure you choose products carefully. Be extremely wary of baby shampoos as some of these are not pH-balanced and are formulated for scalp care rather than for nourishing and cleansing the hair.

dandruff shampoos

Dandruff shampoos have changed dramatically in the past few years. Coal tar, the traditional dandruff cure, has been replaced by new wonder ingredients such as piroctone olamine. The shampoo acts as an exfoliant, as in skincare, to help shed the surplus cells. The best anti-dandruff shampoos include tea tree oil, a natural antiseptic that will not overdry the scalp or damage the hair.

frequently asked questions

Q Is shampooing regularly bad for your hair and will it fade colour?

A No, as long as you use good products that are pH-balanced and contain conditioning agents to seal the cuticle and lock in any colour.

Q Why does my hair feel greasy and my scalp dry after shampooing?

A This comes from not rinsing products away thoroughly. Always rinse the hair until it feels 'squeaky clean' to the touch.

Q Do shampoos, conditioners and styling products cause build-up and if so, what can be done?

A Some products' ingredients can cause a build-up or intolerance. This can be prevented by using a detoxifying shampoo every two weeks, which will also cleanse the hair generally from outside pollution.

the five-step shampoo

1 Thoroughly drench the hair for 30 to 60 seconds before you apply shampoo – you'll need less product and washing will be easier on the hair. Rub a little shampoo between the palms of your hands before smoothing it over the surface of the hair.

2 Gently massage the head, but do not rough up the hair or pull long hair up onto the scalp – it only causes tangles. Long hair will be cleansed as the shampoo washes out with the water.

3 When massaging, use the tips of your fingers, not the palms of your hands. This helps stimulate the scalp and stops you from roughing up the cuticle.

4 Rinse, rinse and rinse again. Poor rinsing results in dull hair and a flaky scalp, caused by dry soap flakes. Finish with an ice-cold rinse. It will close the cuticle and stimulate the scalp, ensuring healthy growth and extra shine.

5 To towel-dry, squeeze and pat the hair dry. Do not rub it too vigorously with the towel as it will rub the hair cuticle up the wrong way.

conditioners

There is much more to conditioners than just their moisturizing ingredients: laws of physics come into play each time you apply one. The positively charged polymers of small and large cationic molecules in the conditioning agents are attracted to and attach themselves to the negatively charged, damaged areas of your hair. In this way, each hair shaft is coated with protective binding and moisturizing ingredients, so conditioners can actually help repair weakened hair. As skincare formulations have become more advanced, so, too, have haircare products, enabling the ingredients to penetrate much deeper into the hair shaft, leaving hair better conditioned and feeling lighter.

hair masks

Deep conditioning treatments and hair masks work on the same principle as everyday conditioners, but because they are left on the hair for longer, they have more time to penetrate the hair shaft. The ingredients are easily absorbed by the hair, so there is no need to leave the treatment on for longer than the recommended time. Use an intensive conditioner or hair mask once a week for super-glossy hair, especially if your tresses are prone to dryness.

leave-in conditioners

These are designed to condition and add shine but do not leave the hair lank which makes them ideal for people with fine, flyaway or difficult-to-manage hair. They are best applied away from the roots.

conditioning tips

Identify your requirements when choosing a conditioner to suit your hair and scalp type, but remember its limitations. No conditioner can replace essential nutrients that are lacking in your diet.

Always read the manufacturer's notes. These provide much more information than ever before, so you shouldn't make the wrong choice.

Once you have applied a hair mask, cover your hair, either with silver foil or clingfilm (saranwrap), both of which lock in the heat and enable the product to penetrate deeper (heat will open the cuticle wider).

Alternatively, drench a towel with hot water and wrap it around your head – you have the bonus of extra heat and the steam will stop the hair drying.

When you rinse off conditioner, finish with a cold blast of water which will close the cuticle, leaving hair glossy and shiny. It will also stimulate blood flow to the scalp, encouraging healthy hair growth.

Key ingredients to look out for in your miracle in a bottle: wheatgerm oil, a natural moisturizer; green tea extract, which helps to retain moisture; and provitamin B5, which enhances gloss.

product power

Hair without styling product is like a sandwich without filling; it's the best way to get the most out of your locks. To maintain tip-top condition, use products that are specially formulated for your hair type and that correspond with your shampoo and conditioner. Avoid sticky products, as these tend to create build-up and can ruin the condition and health of your hair. Also, don't overload your hair – it may lose volume and look lank. Forget old myths about styling products; they have improved dramatically in recent years to give added manageability and the control you need to create certain looks. Try out as many products as you can to see which you like, and ask your stylist for advice.

mousse

The light, airy consistency of mousse makes it easy to distribute evenly. The hold factor depends on the resin content – more resins means more lift and hold.

thickening and volumizing sprays

Like mousses, styling sprays use flexible resins to give body and volume. They give an even coverage and tend to be softer and lighter than mousse; the spray application means it can be directed to specific areas, such as a fringe (bangs) or the roots. Both sprays and mousses help combat static. Styling spray is ideal to use on wet hair or as an instant pick-me-up between washes to give great shape and renewed gloss and bounce. It leaves hair looking natural and protects it from heat-styling damage.

gels

These are used to sculpt a style and contain water-soluble resins and silicones that give a firm hold. Depending on the ratio of water to oil in the formula, gels can vary in consistency from ones that set hard after application to those that keep a wet look.

wax

Originally used in Afro haircare, waxes (or pomades) became the hair gels of the 1990s. Used sparingly, waxes (which contain petroleum jelly) give shine and hold down errant strands by virtue of their adhesive consistency.

serum

The latest hair styling innovation is a volatile silicone which imparts brilliant shine to hair with none of the heaviness of wax. It must be used very sparingly, otherwise hair looks oily. The spray versions tend to be heavier and can't be controlled as well as pump-action serums.

straighteners

These temporarily close down the cuticle to achieve a smooth, sleek finish. Use one in conjunction with a straightening blow-dry (see page 63) and Jennifer Aniston's look could be yours.

always read the label

There are key ingredients to look out for when choosing the right products for your hair type. There is no need to be blinded by science for a moment longer – all will be revealed:

Amino acids act as humectants, drawing moisture into the hair.

Cationic ingredients are positively charged molecules (usually polymers) that are attracted to damaged areas of the hair shaft and lock on to smooth and repair.

Green tea extract is an antioxidant that combats free radical damage and improves hair health.

Panthenol or Provitamin B5 penetrates the hair shaft to improve strength, moisture and shine.

Polymers give bounce and manageability. Water-soluble silicones and dimethicones coat the hair to smooth the cuticle and add shine.

Vitamin E, or tocopherol, is a protective antioxidant that slows down oxidation caused by pollution, smoking, chlorine and UV exposure.

Wheatgerm oil moisturizes the hair and also decreases static.

brushwork

It seems such a simple and obvious thing – using the right tool for the job – and yet few do it. The choice of brush can affect how fast your hair dries, how smooth it is and how much volume you can create. Good-quality bristles protect hair from splitting and stretching, making styling and combing easier and painless, while poor-quality brushes and combs will scratch the scalp and damage the hair shaft. When choosing a brush, always check that the teeth and bristles are smooth.

paddle brush

Broad and rectangular, it smooths hair and works best on long, straight styles. The rubber cushioning on the paddle ensures extra-smooth, static-free hair.

roller and curling brushes

Used with a hairdryer, roller and curling brushes become mobile curlers and achieve volume. Some have a metal barrel that conducts heat from the dryer to reduce drying times. These can be detached from the handle to form a roller, which is ideal for creating long-lasting volume. If your hair has a tendency to be static, then lightly spray the metal barrel with hairspray.

volumizing brushes

These are the ones with an 'open' head and fewer bristles or teeth than most other brushes. The holes work like air vents to circulate warm air from a hairdryer and increase volume and bounce.

smoothing brushes

An essential day-to-day brush that often has a rubber cushion holding the bristles, helping to counter static electricity. It is good to have a mix of natural and nylon bristles – nylon will grip, while natural will smooth.

tail combs

Used for sectioning hair when blow-drying or setting, they are the only way to create a perfect parting.

fork combs

These 'open' up curls and separate kinky, wavy hair.

fine and medium combs

Both of these are used for backcombing and delicate detangling, but are best used by a hairdresser.

wide-tooth combs

Use these to comb conditioner through wet hair.

brushstrokes

Hair is elastic to some extent, but harsh brushing will overstretch and ultimately break the hair.

1 Always brush your hair before shampooing to massage the scalp, help loosen dead skin cells and detangle any knots (the hair becomes more fragile and thus more difficult to detangle when wet).

2 Always brush from the tips up, not from the roots down. This is the best way to detangle hair.

3 To remove a tangle, comb from the base of the tangle to hair tips, working upwards slowly.

4 Once hair is tangle-free, brush from the roots to the tips to distribute sebum along the hair shaft and increase its natural shine.

5 Ignore the '100 brushstrokes a day' maxim. Too much brushing will overstimulate sebum production and increase the chances of oily hair, breakages and split ends. In the Victorian times when this old-wives' tale was coined, 100 strokes a day was a good way of preventing hair lice from multiplying because it destroyed the eggs and damaged the insects. Yuck! Times have changed and so should our grooming habits. Rapunzel had more time on her hands than you.

6 Keep brushes and combs clean and free from stray hairs and product build-up. Add a little shampoo to lukewarm water and soak them for about five minutes, then leave to dry naturally.

inside, outside

In a perfect world we would all be calm, collected and look the picture of health. Unfortunately, though, all too often we are subject to stress, but how we deal with it determines how well we cope and, ultimately, how good we look. Taking supplements, exercising and allowing time to eat well, sleep well and relax will not make your life go more smoothly, but it will give your inner resources an extra boost that will help you manage stress and still have enough energy left to keep your inner light shining brightly.

expect the unexpected

From relatively minor disruptions like the washing machine flooding to more serious problems of health and demands from your work and family, life is full of situations beyond our control. Inevitably, this means we often have to change the best-laid plans at the last moment and adapt accordingly. When we are fit and healthy we are more able to deal with problems and to respond more effectively to them.

don't be too harsh on yourself

Good habits are easy to break and no one is immune to temptation. If your willpower isn't as strong as you'd like, maybe you are expecting too much of yourself. Reconsider your goals. Few people manage to eat a perfectly balanced diet or keep up an exercise routine all of the time.

learn to compromise

We all lead busy, busy lives and free time has become a luxury. If a few microwave meals are a way of spending precious time with your family, then so be it. But you don't have time to relax? You don't have to be in a yoga class to practise slow, deep breathing – do it while driving home in your car or while sitting on the bus.

get as much help as you can

Develop a support system of your favourite products, dietary supplements and pampering treats that you can use to nurture your sense of wellbeing. Keep to hand a list of the numbers of good health, beauty and alternative therapists so that booking a reflexology appointment becomes as easy as dialling out for a takeaway.

stressed hair

When you are worried and stressed, the first part of the body to become tense is the shoulders. When the neck and shoulders are constricted, the supply of oxygen and blood to the scalp is inhibited. Inevitably, your hair becomes stressed, too, and the signs are a flaky scalp, dull hair and, eventually, hair loss. When you are stressed, your nails and hair are the first to be ignored by your body's natural vitamin distribution process – and this is also true for pregnant women. It is absolutely essential to replace lost minerals and vitamins, both internally and externally.

1 Massage the scalp and learn to relax. It relieves tension and increases blood flow which nourishes the root and hair follicle. Gently work your fingers around your head, massaging all the time. Start at the perimeter of the head and work inwards, making sure your fingers never leave the scalp.

2 A flaky scalp can be due to dehydration – especially after too much alcohol – so take a bath to unwind, rather than reaching for the wine bottle, and always drink at least eight large glasses of water every day.

3 Think about supplementing your diet with vitamins and minerals.

4 Eat your greens. Green vegetables have a high iron content that will encourage the growth of healthy hair.

5 Eat oily fish. The oils encourage the flow of sebum, thus giving flexibility to the hair.

6 Essential oils are good for wellbeing and can also benefit the scalp and hair when a few drops are diluted in vegetable oil or warm water. Rose absolut is moisturizing; tea tree and eucalyptus have antiseptic properties which are soothing for a dry, tight scalp; and lavender is supremely relaxing.

Having spent the night on a mattress on Polly's floor, Chrissie feels underwhelmed, jet-lagged and out of sorts. She didn't get the red-carpet treatment she'd been expecting – her sleeping arrangements left a lot to be desired and where was she meant to be hanging up her (extensive) wardrobe? Standing in the bathroom under the glare of a very unflattering light, she realizes that she is experiencing the mother of all bad-hair days. Chrissie's fine flyaway locks are

... chrissie's frazzled-hair crisis

looking fluffy, fuzzy and lank. Her job as beauty therapist on Virtual Airlines has caused big problems on the static front. All those long, carpeted corridors at the airport, the nylon upholstery and the fetching beret she's forced to wear ensure that sparks fly every time she brushes her hair. It's no wonder she's failed to pull the handsome dot.com entrepreneur who commutes to New York every week; each time she gives him a back massage he complains of static shocks. And now this. She looks like a cross between an ageing rock star and Dougal from *The Magic Roundabout*. Working frantically through the contents of the bathroom cabinet, she experiments with every hair product she can lay her hands on in an attempt to groom her sorry, straggling strands – but to no avail. It finally dawns on Chrissie that no amount of serum is going to solve her hair crisis. What her stressed-out mane really needs is some back-to-basic haircare – the magic H_2O (at least 1 litre a day) and some dietary supplements like vitamins B and C (a balanced diet is not one of Chrissie's strong points).

fringe benefits

The debate about whether or not to take supplements is on-going. Many doctors and dieticians believe that a balanced diet, containing plenty of fresh fruit and vegetables, should provide all the nutrients the body needs to function efficiently and at its optimum. However, the lifestyle that many of us lead means that we are frequently under stress and exposed to toxins – both from an intake of caffeine, nicotine, alcohol and overprocessed food, and also from ultraviolet rays, pollution and radiation from office equipment – which can deplete our bodies' stores of essential nutrients.

supplements for hair, skin and nails

Beta-carotene is an antioxidant that is converted in the body to form vitamin A.

Omega-3 provides essential fatty acids.

Starflower oil is a rich source of an essential fatty acid, gamma linolenic acid (GLA), which acts as a building block for healthy skin and hormone balance.

Selenium is a mineral needed for the action of many antioxidant enzymes.

Vitamin B complex promotes healthy hair and skin and supports the central nervous system.

Vitamin C is an antioxidant that destroys harmful free radicals caused by pollution.

Zinc is a mineral that is essential for the proper functioning of over 100 enzymes.

warning

Supplements are virtually non-toxic, so there is no real safety issue. A good multivitamin, multimineral and an antioxidant formula is ideal, but if in doubt, ask a doctor, dietician or pharmacist for advice and always follow the manufacturer's dosage instructions. If you are experiencing any serious problems with your hair, consult a doctor for advice.

supplements for stress

Beta-carotene, selenium and vitamins C and E with zinc work together as antioxidants to disarm damaging free radicals caused by stress.

Bilberry helps prevent the premature death of body cells.

Calcium and magnesium deficiencies are common in highly stressed individuals and can result in anxiety, fear and even hallucinations.

Dong quai supports the kidneys, central nervous system and the adrenal glands, which are among the most susceptible organs to stress.

Gamma-aminobutric acid (GABA) acts as a tranquillizer and is important for proper brain function.

Gingko biloba aids brain function and circulation.

Hops help to ease nervousness, restlessness and stress, and also decrease the desire for alcohol.

Kava kava relaxes the mind as well as the body.

L-Tyrosine is an effective sleeping aid, which is also good for depression.

Valerian is another powerful sleeping aid when taken at bedtime and it also helps ease stress-related headaches.

Vitamin B complex, plus extra vitamin B6 (pyridoxine), B12 and B5 (panothenic acid) are necessary for health and the proper functioning of the nervous system; B5, in particular, is an anti-stress vitamin needed by the thymus gland.

Vitamin C with bioflavonoids is essential for the functioning of the adrenal gland, which produces anti-stress hormones.

your hair talks

chrissie comes to town

'I can't tell you how thrilled I am to be here,' said Chrissie, gliding elegantly into the sitting room, bare-footed and bare-legged, save for a silver chain around her ankle that jangled as she moved. The girls were lined up on the (once) cream-coloured sofa, marvelling at how glamorous their new house guest looked. Despite the fact that it was Sunday morning, Chrissie was wearing full make-up, artfully contrived to look as if she was wearing none at all.

'So I've brought each of you a little present from the Big Apple,' she was saying, dipping into a big honey-coloured leather bag that Jaz instantly recognized as a designer label that you had to join a 12-month waiting-list to own. 'For Polly, my gracious hostess … something sexy to go under all those deathly boring navy-blue suits that you have to wear to work.' Chrissie handed over a little parcel of shell-pink tissue paper containing a scarlet silk camisole with black lace trim. 'I thought it might spice things up a little with Harry,' she added. Polly blushed the same colour as the camisole. It would take more than this to spice things up with Harry, her boyfriend since college. He was a nice enough bloke, but these days he seemed to get more turned on by share prices than by Polly's choice of lingerie. Their relationship had gone a little flat, to say the least. It was a good job that she had flirtatious e-mails from her colleague in New York to look forward to. At least 'cyber-Simon', as she called him, was adding a little fizz to her life. 'And for you, Kate … a new cellulite cream,' Chrissie was saying. 'I've heard

from girlfriends who have cellulite that it really works.' Kate glowered as Chrissie handed over the tube of Fat-busting Miracle Lotion. Jaz, meanwhile, was thrilled with her set of brain-boosting nail polishes containing ginkgo biloba – 'absorbed through the nail bed to improve brain function' – and oblivious to the implied insult. 'And Laura, I think this scent is just the ticket for you. It smells … well, very feminine,' said Chrissie, in what was clearly a dig at Laura's tomboy style. Laura, who never wore perfume, stifled the urge to laugh as she eyed the blurb on the label: 'Fatal: The scent that spells instant attraction'. Love her or loathe her – and Laura hadn't made her mind up yet – there was no denying that Chrissie was a blast.

'Now girls, the good news is that Steve, the record producer I told you about, has invited me to the opening of Shaft, a new bar in Soho, on Saturday night,' Chrissie continued, 'and I've managed to get you all on the guest list.'

'Thanks, but no thanks. I've already got plans,' lied Kate, who would rather boil in oil than spend an evening with Chrissie.

'Count me in,' declared Jaz enthusiastically (she was already painting her toenails orange).

'I'm game,' said Laura. 'What about you, Pol?'

'I'd love to, but I'm flying to New York on Saturday afternoon for business and I'll be away for the rest of the week,' replied Polly, who could hardly contain her excitement at the prospect of finally meeting Simon, her sexy (she hoped) cyber-suitor.

cut it

There are no limitations to your choice of style or cut. Modern fashion and beauty tells us that anything goes: all that matters is that you feel happy and confident with your look. If you have a long, sloping jaw, traditional thinking would tell you to avoid a short gamine cut, but if you like it and have the confidence to wear it, the chances are you will pull it off beautifully. Just look at all those quirky models who don't fit the perfectly proportioned, blonde-haired, blue-eyed aesthetic. But if you don't feel brave enough to throw caution to the wind, here are few guidelines that will guarantee that a cut suits your face and flatters your features in a more classical manner.

face shape

The best way to determine your face shape is by doing the mirror trick (see page 36). Alternatively, get a photo taken or rely on your hairdresser to define your profile. Certain features can be minimized or emphasized by a hairstyle. A prominent nose or chin can be countered by a fringe (bangs). An angular jawbone means you can wear gamine Audrey Hepburn cuts and crops, while a long, sloping jawbone doesn't always work with short hair.

Remember that your face shape changes with age. Your jaw will inevitably grow less defined and your complexion less radiant and smooth as you grow older. The good news is that a clever cut and colour can make you look younger and feel better. Don't get stuck in a rut, repeating the same hairstyle time and time again, keep moving with the times. After all, what suits you at 18 is unlikely to look good when you are 30. Nothing will date you faster than make-up and a haircut, and yet nothing is quite so simple to change.

oval face

This classic shape can take any look. With this in mind, use your hairstyle to create an illusion of the perfect oval by balancing out the proportions.

heart-shaped

The narrowing of the face can be countered with the extra volume of a layered bob, which flicks outwards at chin level.

square face

Soften up the edges with a style that breaks up the symmetry. Play with off-centre partings, graduated layers and soft curls.

round face

Soft, feathery cuts with layers coming forward onto the face look stylish and sophisticated and also slim down a fuller face.

long face

A fringe (bangs) disguises a long forehead, while a chin- or shoulder- length style adds volume and broadens the face.

parting company

Creating a new parting is the quickest and cheapest way to update a style and change your look and face shape. Each season, one type of parting dominates the fashion shows – from the zigzag to the deep, side parting just above the ear. For a long time only centre partings would do. Use a tail comb to experiment. Hold it by the teeth at a low angle and use the handle to part the hair. Keep the tip in contact with the scalp to get the most control.

body proportion

As well as considering your hair type and face shape, a good hairdresser will also take into account your body shape, proportions and size when consulting you about a restyle. This is why it is important that he or she sees you to discuss your ideas before you are sitting in a chair, shrouded in a gown and with your hair wrapped up in a towel on top of your head.

Very long, flowing hair on a short body frame will foreshorten the body even more; conversely, a short, gamine crop will not work well on a body that is broad-framed and tall. Big-volume curly shoulder-length hair on a short, plump torso will just accentuate width; while a short, spiky cut on a tall person can be intimidating.

how to determine face shape

1 Stand in front of your mirror, face on.

2 Using your hands, pull all your hair right away from your face.

3 Take a lipstick (not your favourite) and, at arm's length, draw around the outline of your face on the mirror.

4 Like it or not, what you are left with is your face shape.

Laura is quite the antithesis of Jaz. That's not to say she doesn't care about her image – she always manages to look effortlessly cool – she just can't be doing with Jaz's overwhelming 'girliness'. Listening to her and

… laura's restyle

Chrissie prattle on last night about the best pink nail polish and where to buy the prettiest handkerchief tops had almost driven her to commit a violent act. Laura has a much more pragmatic approach to beauty. She loves to work out and has had the same boyish crop – quick to wash and dry after her gym sessions – since she started at university in Manchester, which is well over five years ago now. She knows that it's definitely time

for a restyle (her mind was well and truly made up when she heard someone refer to her as 'him' – she did have her back turned, but nevertheless it was not a moment she ever wants to revisit). Laura books up an appointment with her hairstylist who, after a lengthy discussion – after all, this is not a decision to be taken lightly – enthusiastically cuts and restyles her hair. The end result gives her more height on the crown, a soft, wispy fringe

(bangs) on her forehead and light flick-outs on the nape of her neck. The crowning glory, however, is that this new style disguises her large forehead and shortens her long face (not that she would ever admit to minding about these features) – amazing how a cut can change the shape of your face. Laura strides out of the salon with a spring in her step, secretly hoping that the assistant producer in Current Affairs will sit up and take notice.

the cutting edge

A good haircut should make you feel fantastic. It should increase your confidence, make you feel sexy, taller, slimmer, more powerful, and, most importantly, it should reflect your personality. Styled in the right way, a haircut can even act as an instant 'facelift', helping to detract attention from areas of the face that show signs of ageing and, instead, highlight your most flattering features, perhaps great bone structure or beautiful eyes. A good cut will give your entire look a new lease of life – while a little colour on your tresses will make it look thicker and glossier, too (see page 44). Hair is usually the first thing to be altered when a woman is making a major life change – perhaps a new career direction or at the beginning (or end) of a relationship. A visit to the hairdresser's for a spot of pampering or reinvention is also a sure-fire way to lift a bad mood. Once you've found the right hairstyle, everything else falls into place. Whatever the reason and whatever the style, always have a trim every six weeks to avoid split ends and help maintain condition and manageability.

cutting considerations

There are three essential points to consider before embarking on any change of image:

1 Be realistic. How much time do you really want to spend on your hair every day? Also, how much time have you realistically got? If you choose a style that requires time you are not happy to put in, you will never get the look you want.

2 Straight, curly, dark or blonde, wavy or wispy, make the most of what you've got. Hair always looks its best when it is in fabulous condition and has a fantastic cut.

3 Use your ammunition! Products are essential daily tools for achieving gloss, body and manageability on all hair types. Experiment a little and learn which products suit your hair best and how to use them.

the long and the short of it

Long, romantic, tumbling tresses remain a classic look and a favourite with the opposite sex. To counter the hippie 'curtain' effect and make your hair seem less heavy, as well as keep locks in excellent condition, go for a layered cut. This will add shape around your face to give a defined and confident style. With well-shaped layers, hair will not fall too heavily across the face. But be warned: there's nothing worse than straggly, uncared-for, 'rat tail' hair snaking down your back, so don't bother growing it if you don't want to spend time brushing, washing, drying and styling it.

With its mix of modernity and femininity, short hair can be extremely sexy. It is a great option for women who want a strong, feminine image, a personal signature, yet a low-maintenance style. Short, sassy, sexy styles are on the increase – think Meg Ryan, Gwyneth Paltrow and Cameron Diaz. Casual or glamorous, layers help to define texture and volume, giving the hair greater depth and making styling simple.

going for the chop

Ultimately, whether you opt for a long or short style, determining your face shape, hair type and texture will help you to find the most flattering cut for you. Once you have this basic information to work with, you can then adapt catwalk styles or ideas from the pages of beauty magazines to create an individual look. The key thing to remember is that the face shape should trigger off the hairstyle. In the same way as a beautiful frame enhances a picture, if you've got the right hairstyle for your face shape, then your whole face will look prettier and fresher, your eyes will stand out and your good features will be emphasized. Enjoy your hair's own unique style and, with the advice of your hairdresser, select a style to enhance what you've already got. If you try to alter your natural hair too much, you may end up compromising on the condition of your hair and become a slave to a high-maintenance look in the process.

your hairdresser

Finding a hairstylist with whom you 'click' is like any other relationship – although it's unlikely you'd ask a friend to make you look and feel like a groovier version of your favourite actress. You need chemistry, you need trust and you need to be able to convey your ideas in such a way that they can be easily interpreted. If you are considering a radical cut but don't have a hairdresser you trust, book in a few blow-drys at different salons. Mention your ideas to the stylist looking after you and decide with whom you feel most at ease. All good salons offer a free consultation, but having a blow-dry will allow you to experience how a stylist works, rather than just listen to their suggestions. Apart from anything else, visiting a salon should be a pleasurable experience. You want to feel pampered and relaxed, confident in the knowledge that when you walk out you are going to look and feel like a million dollars, not nervous and edgy, wishing you'd brought a paper bag with you.

Recommendations from friends are a good way of finding a reputable stylist, but we are all subjective in our choices, and one person's dream stylist could be another's idea of hell. If you see someone with a haircut you like, ask them who did it. After all, you wouldn't hesitate to question where someone got their stunning kitten heels that you liked the look of, now would you?

the consultation

Taking along a picture of a cut or colour you like is a good starting point and avoids confusion. Compile a 'look book' – a scrapbook or folder where you keep tear sheets from magazines of styles you like, as well as photographs of yourself when you had a particularly good cut or colour. It's also useful to show your stylist pictures of looks that you really dislike. A picture is a good way of understanding one another's vocabulary – for you, titian may mean coppery golden tints; for your stylist it may mean gingery red tones. However, do not expect to look like the person in the picture – sadly for us, there is only one Rachel, one Meg and one Gwyneth.

reworkings and rewards

If you don't like a cut or style, be honest and tell your stylist. They would much prefer to rework it and sort it out for you, rather than have you leave disappointed. Conversely, if you really like a cut or receive a lot of compliments on a style, give the stylist that feedback. Everyone responds to praise and likes to know when a cut or style performs well.

If you are happy with the stylist's work, then tip, but don't feel uneasy if you can't afford to tip heftily. Ask any hairdresser and they are thrilled if they receive a thank-you card or see a customer leave the salon looking genuinely happy. Equally, if you buy a bottle of the shampoo, conditioner or styling product that your stylist has used, this indicates that you want to re-create the look again at home.

hairdressers' translation service

Choppy This is the result when hair has been cut using a texturizing method – for example, razor-cutting to give a 'choppy finish'.

Feathery Using a razor to cut hair instead of scissors. This creates a much more random finish, leaving the hair more dishevelled and giving that lived-in look.

Flick-outs This involves blow-drying the hair so that it flicks outwards at the ends to create volume and width, instead of blow-drying the hair under, which is a more traditional look.

Texturizing A method of cutting using tools such as a razor, clippers or texturizing scissors. These are like ordinary cutting scissors, but one blade is serrated, enabling the stylist to reduce weight evenly throughout the cut.

Volume To build hair and add life, volume can be temporary or permanent.

... polly's hair therapy

Chrissie's arrival at the house has precipitated a bit of a *crise* in Polly's life. She takes one look at Chrissie's tardis-like suitcase – the contents of which are now strewn across her bedroom floor – and can't help but compare her own black, grey and navy blue power suits and boring black and white basics with Chrissie's endless supply of skimpy tops in every shade of pink and purple, bead-fringed capri pants and flirty, diaphanous skirts. And was that a diamanté, heart-shaped body jewel stuck to her sensible beige carpet? Polly decides there is nothing else for it but to book a day at her favourite hair and beauty spa for a bit of top-to-toe pampering. She's been 'seeing' Charles for years – he always has a knack of understanding exactly what she wants, and has a chair-side manner to die for – not to mention the great haircuts. After lots of hair chat (so much better than therapy), Polly decides to have her shoulder-length blonde hair lightly layered, which will soften her face and groove up her look. Best of all, it can be zooped up with products for that hip rock-chick look – although the latter probably won't go down too well with the suits on the top floor at work! Polly feels fantastic. Harry won't recognize her – on second thoughts, he probably won't even notice.

colour coding

Colour adds sheen, gloss, texture, thickness, depth and life to your hair and can be used either to enhance your natural hair colour or to explore a different side of your personality and change your image. Never be afraid to experiment, especially when you have a trusted stylist with whom you feel safe enough to be a little more daring. A good colourist will work with your skin tone and personality to create an effect that suits your style and boosts your confidence.

hue are you?

An experienced colourist is able to determine quickly whether you are a 'whisper', 'talk' or 'scream' type of customer – in other words, whether you would be more comfortable with a few lowlights in your mousey brown hair or whether you are an extrovert who will feel perfectly at ease with a white-blonde crop. Often a customer profile questionnaire is used as part of a two-way discussion between stylist and customer to establish which colours will go best with your personality, as well as which will suit your complexion.

the home colour zone

Use the colour chart on pages 48–9 to work out whether you are a 'warm' or 'cool' customer. This will help you determine which hair colours will best enhance your skin tone (see right).

1 Stand in front of a mirror in good (preferably natural) light, holding the colour chart just underneath your chin.

2 Slowly move it from left to right and back again and observe which colour tones are the most flattering to your complexion.

3 Repeat the process a few times and ask the opinion of a friend.

HAIR SNIP

MODERN HAIR COLORANTS ARE ENRICHED WITH CONDITIONING INGREDIENTS, SO YOU CAN ENHANCE YOUR NATURAL COLOUR WITHOUT DAMAGING THE HEALTH OF YOUR TRESSES. HOWEVER, ANY CHEMICAL TREATMENT MEANS THAT THE HAIR WILL REQUIRE GENTLE HANDLING. USE EXTRA-NOURISHING CONDITIONERS AND APPLY A HYDRATING MASK ONCE A WEEK TO REPLENISH MOISTURE. AVOID HOT-OIL TREATMENTS AS THEY TEND TO STRIP OUT COLOUR.

natural mixes

The colour of your hair should be from the same family (warm or cool) as your skin tone. If you have very pale skin, any colour will look good; if you have pink skin, avoid reds and warm golds; if your skin has yellow tones, favour deep reds and avoid golds; those with black or olive skin should stay dark, adding richness and depth with lowlights. Use the following guide to help determine what hair colour will best suit your complexion and colouring, or try on wigs or hairpieces.

warm

Eyes: brown, hazel, green or dark brown.

Skin: freckles, golden beige, bronze or golden brown.

Hair: golden or strawberry blonde, golden brown or auburn, chestnut or dark brown.

cool

Eyes: grey-blue, grey-brown or rose-brown.

Skin: beige, rose-brown or cocoa.

Hair: ash blonde, ash brown, beige blonde, black, burgundy or plum.

colour glossary

cool

semi-permanent colour

These are vegetable-based dyes that penetrate slightly into the hair, then simply wash away. They last for about 12 washes. You can go only darker or warmer than your natural colour.

highlights

With highlighting, strands of hair are placed in foils and dyed a lighter shade than your natural colour. Bold strands create a strong effect, while fine pieces give a more natural look. As the dye is permanent, the roots will need retouching when the highlights grow out.

permanent colour

These dyes can improve the condition of the hair while adding colour. You can go lighter, darker or change the tone completely. The colour does not appear artificial, no matter how vivid the tone. This process can be carried out as a full head or as pieces of colour.

lowlights

With lowlights, strands of hair are placed in foils and dyed a darker shade than your natural hair colour. The dye is permanent. This is a very good method of adding depth and tone to dull hair – you can be as subtle or as bright as you want.

colour wash

Change your look for the weekend with a colour wash. This temporary colour is available as a coloured mousse or setting lotion and will last for just one wash. Also known as vegetable colours, these are excellent for refreshing faded colour and can be used as a conditioning treatment.

tone on tone

This technique blends white hair and adds tone and shine. It will not lighten hair, but gives it sheen and life. Tone-on-tone lasts between four and six weeks. This can also be used within creative-colour techniques to give subtle depth and evenness.

shading

Two or three shades of colour are applied to each 'slice' of hair. Semi-permanent colour can be used for a subtle look; tone-on-tone for visible colour; and permanent colour for a dramatic effect. This is a really good technique for thickening fine hair, as the multi-colour shading gives depth.

chunky lights

Normally applied on the top of the head and around the face, colour is added to wide-woven pieces of hair. Softer or stronger colours can be used to create different effects. This technique is best when slightly contrasting colours are used, as it will make the colour stand out.

bleaching

This technique is used to lighten hair or to create results that cannot be achieved with high-lift tint. Bleaching agents lighten the pigments of the hair and rinsing stops the process at the required shade. It's a job best left to the experts, as toning is a major part of this process.

duo/trio colour

A creative technique using tone-on-tone colour, which can be semi-permanent or permanent. Colour is applied in two sections to cover the whole head and can be subtle or dramatically different. Duo colour means two colours only; trio is three colours only.

waxes and pomades

Colour waxes or pomades are a totally temporary colouring method, ideal for those who like to go wild at the weekend but have to look smart during the week. It is applied after the hair has been dried and styled to give a dramatic look. If you have very blonde or bleached hair, do a test strand to make sure it doesn't stain the hair and will wash out.

tonal blast

The tips of the hair are first lightened and then tone-on-tone colour is applied. The lightened pieces of hair will show the tone more dramatically. This colour adds definition to shorter haircuts and works best when stronger colours, such as reds and coppers, are used.

warm

... jaz's creative-colour experience

Jaz's girlfriend, Vicci, whose passion for fashion equals Jaz's, has a younger sister who's a junior stylist at one of London's top salons. She's told them they're looking for models for creative colouring and, since Jaz has such great hair, would she be up for it? Stupid question! Jaz is there as quick as you can say highlights. She's been chosen for tie-dyeing – cool. What amazing timing with this party coming up at Shaft with Chrissie and the

girls. She really wants to look hot – apparently it's going to be packed with movers and shakers from the media and the fashion pack. Jaz can hardly contain her excitement, which is not quite so cool, she realizes. While the hairstylist divides her hair into sections, she pictures herself working the room at Shaft and holding court, with a hip designer hanging on to her every word. These happy thoughts are interrupted by a serious style

issue. What shade of nail polish will look best with her fuchsia-pink, bias-cut slip dress? Before she knows it (amazing how absorbing such matters can be), her hair has been sectioned with hair bands, scrunched up, coloured, washed and blow-dried. And – hey presto – her dark black, glossy locks are now mottled with variegated shades of red. Fab – it's just like the skirt she bought last weekend from Portobello market. Love it!

colouring tips

lighten up, but **not** at home

Attempting to lighten your hair yourself, using home-made preparations, lemon juice or – horror – bleach, is an extremely precarious business. Do without that must-have pair of feathered mules if need be, but leave your highlighting to the professionals. If you don't, you'll probably end up having to visit the salon anyway for a rescue job.

troubleshooting

If your hair has been coloured in a salon and you are unhappy with the end result, talk to your hairdresser; there are several things they can do. Colour can be masked or returned to your natural shade. Brassy or yellow bleached hair can be toned down with silvery or ashy temporary colour and a tint will also cover bleached hair. A colour stripper or reducer can also be used by your hairdresser to remove permanent tints. Repeated washing will lift semi-permanent colours, but this damages the condition of the hair, so always apply a protein-restructuring mask afterwards.

refresh your tresses

To revive your hair colour, use a colour enhancing shampoo and conditioner once a week. Always follow the manufacturer's instructions and leave them on for the specified time. Minuscule amounts of colour pigment will be deposited on the hair shaft to revitalize and maintain the colour. Vary this treatment with a shampoo and conditioner that has been specially formulated and designed to cope with the changes your hair has undergone.

shampoo/conditioner speak

Shampoos that have been specially formulated for colour-treated hair are designed to condition and cleanse the hair, as well as prevent the colour from fading. Conditioners formulated for colour-treated hair leave a protective film around porous, damaged areas of the hair shaft, helping to lock in the colour pigments and improve the condition of the hair, leaving it stronger and shinier.

don't be dull

If your hair has a tendency to look dull after it has been coloured, a good, quick and very natural treatment is to crack a raw egg onto your head after shampooing and work it through the hair. Leave it for five minutes and then rinse it out thoroughly. Top tip: Use cold or lukewarm water; if the water is too hot you will find that the egg will scramble and it will be difficult to remove. The natural proteins in eggs will leave the hair glossy and full of body.

natural remedy

If you find yourself in a fix without professional products, you can resort to Mother Nature. If your coloured hair has been in the sun and feels brittle and dry, mash up an avocado and work it into your hair after shampooing. Leave it on for at least five minutes to let the moisturizing oils penetrate the hair shaft, then rinse it off thoroughly.

fade out

If you find that your naturally brown hair starts to look dull and faded, steep three tea bags in a large jug of hot water, let it cool down and use it to rinse the hair. The natural dye in tea will even out and enhance the colour of your hair. Similarly, if your naturally blonde hair starts to look dull, rinse it with a solution of camomile tea made as described above. The antioxidant ingredients in the tea will leave your hair fresh, bright and glossy.

chlorine alert

Swimming in chlorinated water can turn bleached or blonde-tinted hair an unsightly shade of green. To prevent this, use products that have been specially designed to protect the hair in chlorinated water, and always rinse your hair immediately after swimming. To restore natural and enhanced blonde hair to its former glory, massage tomato juice into the hair after shampooing; leave for a few minutes and then rinse it out thoroughly. The active ingredients in the tomato juice will neutralize the green colour.

hair to wear

party prep at number 23

Saturday afternoon and very loud disco music was pumping out of the stereo over the non-stop whir of a hairdryer at number 23 Havana Road. There was definite excitement in the air. Chrissie was blow-drying Jaz's hair in the kitchen, Laura had just returned from her Fab Abs class at the gym and Polly was in her bedroom, packing for her trip to New York. In less than 12 hours, she would finally meet cyber-suitor Simon. His last e-mail had been especially flirtatious: 'Don't forget to bring your dancing shoes,' he had written. It usually took Polly 20 minutes tops to pack for a business trip, but today she had dithered for several hours and instead of her usual organized approach, clothes and shoes were strewn Chrissie-style across the bed. Dizzy with excitement, she finally tossed the scarlet camisole, a pair of high heels and a bias-cut slip dress into her case, along with the sensible navy business suits, of course. She jumped guiltily when Kate poked her head around the door to say goodbye, 'I'm off to the hairdressers. Have fun in New York, Pol.'

Kate was glad that she had a hair appointment to go to. Not only was the pounding music driving her mad, but the sight of their house guest running around in an endless selection of tight-fitting clothes – all flat stomach, long legs and sleek blonde hair – really was just too much. Still, it had increased Kate's resolve. After years of flowing, pre-Raphaelite locks and long floral dresses, the time had come to sharpen up her image and start climbing up that career ladder. She was even going to attend a Colour Me Beautiful session at a girlfriend's house that night. Matthew – her handsome boss, the marketing director – wouldn't recognize her on Monday.

At 6 pm Polly's cab arrived. 'Bye girls, I'm off now. Have a great time at the party,' she yelled above the music. Laura was trying to watch a political discussion on television while she waited for Jaz and Chrissie to make their grand entrances. She had been ready for hours, having showered and scrunched some mousse through her hair at the gym. She was pleased with her new, slightly wispier crop, although it'd seemed to have escaped the notice of the assistant producer in Current Affairs. She had no idea what this party would be like, but she'd pushed out the boat and had swapped her uniform of jeans and trainers for a slim-fitting skirt and – hell, it was worth a try – a spritz of 'Fatal'.

Jaz, meanwhile, had pulled out all the stops. She was desperate to wave goodbye to her job as a retail consultant at The Flag and land a plum position with a top designer. This party was the perfect opportunity for career enhancement, since it would be packed with fashionistas. Her new tie-dyed hair and matching red-and-black dip-dyed skirt ought to be enough to get her noticed.

Chrissie was also planning on having a little career advancement of her own. Determined to secure an audition – and a date – with Steve the producer, she had opted for 'result wear'.

Laura and Jaz gasped as she panthered into the living room. Her skin-tight black shell top was practically transparent, her heels as high as the Empire State Building and her fine, flyaway hair looked 'Big' with a capital 'B', thanks to some deft work with her hairdryer and some styling product. 'Let's go, girls,' she cried.

hair-styling

With a few good products and a little practice, anyone should be able to turn a bad-hair day into a good one. Learning how to use styling products effectively and achieving a good blow-dry at home are the first lessons. The critical point is the 'damp to dry' stage when hair has a style 'memory'. If you overdry your hair, spritz it with a little water from a plant mister.

basic blow-dry

1 Gently pat as much moisture away from wet hair as possible using a towel. Rubbing the hair will ruffle the cuticles and causes tangles.

2 Hair loses one-quarter of its elasticity when it is wet, so gently comb it from the tips.

3 Tip your head upside-down and rough-dry your hair with the dryer on medium heat until it is 70 per cent dry. Lift and separate the hair at the roots and through the length with your fingers to create volume.

4 When the hair is still slightly damp, apply the styling product. Then section the back, top, fringe (bangs) and sides with big clips.

5 Starting at the back, unclip and style one section at a time. Use the brushes to lift the hair at the roots, then pull away to dry the length. Spend most effort and time on the front and side sections – once the frame to the face looks good, the rest follows.

6 A fine shot of cool air on the hair, while still under brush control, will set the hair and close the cuticles, giving extra shine.

7 For the finishing touch, add a spot of serum for shine, a little wax to get a choppy look or just a spritz of hairspray to set the style.

HAIR SNIP
ALWAYS RUN THE HAIRDRYER DOWN THE LENGTH OF THE HAIR SHAFT TO KEEP THE CUTICLES LYING FLAT.

TIP YOUR HEAD UPSIDE-DOWN AND SPRAY HAIRSPRAY AT THE ROOTS TO CREATE BIG VOLUME.

tool kit

brushes

Your hairstyle will probably require at least two different brushes, depending on the hair length. One should be a round brush for smoothing or curling and the other a volumizing brush (see page 24).

hairdryer

Choose a hairdryer with a minimum strength of 1500 watts, several heat and force settings and a cold button for finishing.

products

Have to hand the appropriate mousse, gel, serum or styling spray for your particular type of hair and style (see page 23).

comb

A comb is used for careful detangling, sectioning off hair for styling and for creating partings.

clips

These hold sections of hair out of the way while you are blow-drying and styling.

natural drying

1 Start by applying your chosen styling product, spreading it evenly through your hair using your fingers and finishing with a comb.

2 'Mould' your hair into the desired shape before drying it to ensure a perfect finish.

3 Start drying your hair, using your fingers as a brush. This will give maximum lift at the roots.

4 Dry all sections thoroughly and then finish using a light wax.

great curls

1 Apply a styling product that is suitable for your hair type – it is really important to start with a great foundation.

2 Tip your head to one side and, using the bowl of the diffuser, lift the hairdryer up and down into the hair with a gentle movement. Then tip your head to the other side and repeat.

3 When the hair is dry, tip your head forward and carry on with a similar motion. If you find your hair is starting to go fluffy, spritz it with a shine spray.

4 When you have finished all the sections of the hair, gently run a serum evenly through it to create a more defined curl.

straightening

Here are some step-by-step tips for taming your tresses to create bone-straight sleek hair.

1 Start by applying your chosen product evenly through the hair – an anti-frizz serum is ideal.

2 Beginning at the back, use clips to section the hair. Avoid taking too big a section.

3 Using a paddle brush, dry each section in a downwards motion. Start at the roots, taking the brush right through to the ends of the hair. To finish each section, give the hair a blast of cold air.

4 When all the sections of the hair are dry, lightly spray with hairspray to seal the cuticles.

5 Heat the straightening irons and, when they are very hot, run them section by section from the roots to the ends of the hair to ensure Cleopatra-style straight hair. This will seal the cuticles of the hair, leaving it almost impossible for any moisture to penetrate the shaft.

6 To complete the look, spray the hair with a light mist of glossing spray.

HAIR SNIP

IF THERE IS A LOT OF MOISTURE IN THE AIR, OR IT IS VERY HUMID, USE AN ANTI-HUMIDITY SPRAY. THESE CONTAIN ANTI-HUMECTANTS WHICH SEAL THE HAIR AND BLOCK MOISTURE. A LEAVE-IN CONDITIONER WILL ALSO HELP PREVENT YOUR SLEEK LOCKS FROM BECOMING A FRIZZY MESS. ALTERNATIVELY, MIX TWO PARTS OF GEL WITH ONE PART OF SERUM AND APPLY IT TO WET HAIR.

quick fixes

1 If your hair is short, try slicking it back into a sleek crop or simply use pretty pins to decorate it.

2 If your hair is dirty, pin it up. Day-old hair is always easier to put up and will stay in place better than freshly washed hair. Turn unclean hair to your advantage by making a finger-combed ponytail on the crown of your head (avoid too much brushing as this increases the oiliness) and tie it with an elastic. Twist a length of hair around the elastic, fixing it with grips as you go. Let locks of different lengths twist out if they want to; the more effortless the look, the higher the glam factor.

3 If your hair is curly, revitalize it by spritzing it with water and gently scrunching. If it has become frizzy, work a little serum through each tendril, tackling it section by section.

4 If your hair is flat, try a little back-combing to give it lift. Start at the crown and work your way around to the sides. You don't need to backcomb all over, just enough to give a little lift.

5 Do not try to slick back dirty hair with copious amounts of wet-look gel. Although it looks good in magazines, in reality no one is fooled.

6 Never underestimate how long it takes to wash and dry your hair. Forfeit a shampoo for a spot of inventive yet speedy styling.

7 If you are not confident with grips and combs (quick-fix 1), it is better to shower and leave with fresh, clean-smelling but perhaps damp hair than to get frustrated in front of a mirror.

8 Keep an emergency hair kit in the car or office that includes: a brush, a cordless straightener or curling iron, the nearly finished bottles of mousse and serum from home, and a few grips and elastics that can save the day.

9 When you get given another hairdryer for Christmas, take one to the office. It is amazing how many times you get caught in the rain.

10 If your hair is really greasy and you have no time to wash it, apply some dry shampoo or talc close to the roots. Massage it in gently to absorb the excess oil and then brush it out. Or, use cotton wool to dab a little witch hazel onto the roots to absorb any grease.

style-and-go tips

1 To control static, flyaway hair, simply spray a comb with hairspray and gently run it through your locks.

2 Cheap shampoos containing strong detergents will strip your hair of its natural oils and make it seem dull, lank and lifeless.

3 If your hair is very tangled, work it through with a comb first before you begin to use your brush. This will cause as little damage as possible.

4 Keep it cool. Using a hairdryer on a cool setting is good for the scalp, especially if you have greasy hair. Apply too much heat and the scalp will perspire for up to 15 minutes after you've finished drying, causing your hair to drop and lose its shape. It will also activate the oil-producing glands. Whatever your hair type, avoid overdrying, too.

5 Sleep on a satin pillowcase to avoid 'bed-head' hair. In the night your hair will slide gently across it, whereas cotton causes friction which can disrupt the hair cuticles.

6 If, on the other hand, you want to achieve 'bed-head' hair, apply mousse to slightly damp hair before you go to bed. In the morning, simply arrange into place with styling wax or pomade.

7 To keep the hair shaft blunt and prevent split ends, have a trim at least every six weeks.

8 Touch your hair as little as possible after styling it. Otherwise it will lose its shape and body and could become greasy.

9 Simple styles can be energized with temporary colour. Try using hair mascara in bright blue or black for an extra-daring look.

10 To reduce the effects of static hair in the mornings, wrap your hair loosely in a silk headscarf before going to bed. (Probably only worth trying if you sleep alone!)

11 To avoid flat hair, make sure your hair is totally dry when you go to bed. With slightly damp hair, you may well wake up with a frizzy mop, and it's more likely to be flat against your scalp.

12 Two-in-one products can be a great timesaver, but avoid using those that are silicone-based. These build up a coating on the hair which makes it difficult to style.

interview hair

Big hair with lots of root lift was where stylish hair was at in the 1980s – think of the stars of *Dynasty* and *Dallas.* Thankfully, though, these days hair that means business is definitely sleek, easy and under control. The thinking being that if you can't keep your hair under control, how can you possibly be keeping your business under control either? Groomed hair is smart-and-together hair; a sleek ponytail, a smart, short crop or a bob are the perfect styles, and shiny, silky hair in tip-top condition is a must.

It is often quoted that employers decide in the first three minutes into an interview who they are going to employ. To make a good impression, ensure your hair is clean and shiny, as it is an obvious sign that you take care of yourself – the thinking being that if you don't take care of yourself, will you take care of your job? Make sure that your hair is not overly elaborate. If a style looks like it takes an age to create, you will be sending out signals that you will be wasting company time checking your reflection in mirrors. Leave elaborate hairstyles to ladies who lunch, who have nothing more important on their minds than their next Caesar salad. A ponytail can be elegant, but girly styles like plaits and braiding are a no-no if you want to be taken seriously. Depending on the type of business, leave the pink bow and glitter hair slides for the evening. Your Hello Kitty hair accessories won't impress a bank or law firm.

updos

Sleek, chic and giving the appearance of being effortlessly elegant and well-groomed, long hair pinned up in a chignon always means business. Even simpler ponytails can work just as well on hair that is layered or growing out as on straight, one-length hair.

1 Tidy up growing-out layers and feather-cuts by combing through some holding mousse before tying back the hair.

2 Your hairdresser can show you how to attach a hairpiece in the same colour as your own hair to add bulk to a thin ponytail.

3 Avoid tying your hair back towards the crown. Positioned too high, your chic updo will become a cheerleader's ponytail.

4 Keep a hairpiece for ponytails handy on business trips. That way, even if you don't have time to wash your hair, you can tie it back, slick it down and look super-stylish in a moment.

5 Wrap a small strand of hair around the elastic so that it can't be seen and fix it with a grip on the underside. It finishes off the look better than a hair accessory. Alternatively, to make sure your ponytail is really secure, use wet string instead of an elastic to hold it. The string will contract as it dries, fixing the hair in place. As before, wrap a small section of hair around the string to hide it.

6 Slick down wispy bits with a little serum and hairspray to keep the look sleek rather than sporty.

7 If your hair is fine and flyaway, wash it the day before so it's easier to handle and stays in place.

power bobs

The simple bob – with or without a fringe (bangs); curled-up, curled-under or straight; short or long; blunt-cut or wispy – always means business. There is a variation to suit everyone, so talk to your hairdresser about finding the one that suits you. It can be made sleeker or choppier with styling products, depending on your mood. It is the versatility of the bob that keeps it so fresh, even though it has been around since the 1920s.

... kate's take on a power bob

Kate can't bear the thought of looking like a cross between a 1970s throwback from the easy-care perm days and Goldilocks for one minute longer. With her crush on Matthew the marketing director growing more intense by the week, Kate is increasingly interested in how she appears at work. While munching her way through a packet of the latest Crunch biscuits (all in the name of research), she'd read a magazine article entitled confidently 'How to Get Ahead at Work'. Point number three, which was all about image and self-projection, had made quite an impression. With new resolve – a woman with a mission – she hurtles to the hairdresser and demands a power bob (also advised in the very same article). Her patient stylist explains that a classic power bob is a no-no with her hair type; it was never going to look like Uma Thurman's poker-straight 'do' in *Pulp Fiction*. What he can do, though, is give her a sleeker, more groomed look, by taking off some length, adding some layers and generally tidying up her tresses into a bob shape.

Kate starts feeling calmer and her breathing becomes more regulated as she watches herself being transformed into Miss Get Ahead at Work (and, more to the point, Miss How to Get Mr Marketing Director to Look Twice). Her stylist suggests blow-drying her hair straight (the closest she will ever get to a true power bob). Kate can't believe her eyes – she looks like Julia Roberts with sleek hair at the Oscars (sort of). Mr MD – wake up and smell the coffee! For the first time in her life, Kate can't wait to get to work on Monday.

work to play

The invite is for drinks at 7:30, or dinner at 8, yet you know you won't finish work until 6:30 at the earliest. Even if you do get off early, there is no way you can negotiate the cross-town, rush-hour traffic, get changed and get back in time. If you try (and everyone has done it once), you end up frazzled, in a foul temper and 30 minutes late. How much better, then, to make the work-to-play transition in the office or at a nearby gym.

One advantage of choosing a hairstylist near your office is that many salons now offer beauty treatments and have showering facilities available. Build a good relationship with your stylist and you will never have to change at work again. If an invite is sprung on you at the last moment and you have no change of clothes, it is amazing how a professional blow-dry can improve your spirits and your appearance. Your boring suit and white T-shirt suddenly look pared-down and Calvin Klein-ish with an expert coiff. If the salon option is out of the question, opt for one of these styles or try one of the quick fixes on page 64.

twisted sister

1 Start by dividing all of the hair into 5-cm (2-in) square sections. Use sectioning clips to hold them out of the way.

2 Starting at the nape, take each section individually and twist it tightly from the root through to the ends. As you work your way up each section, you'll find that it starts to twist down onto itself. Let this happen until it is sitting on your starting point, then secure it in place with a matt grip.

3 Repeat this, working your way up the head to the crown, until you have twisted each section.

4 Finish by spritzing with a non-aerosol hairspray, which will ensure a strong hold.

glam-hair updo

1 Loosely tie your hair back in a ponytail using a snag-free elastic to maintain a strong hold.

2 Lightly backcomb the ponytail section to create extra volume.

3 Fold sections of the ponytail into the middle of the head, securing them in place with matt grips placed close to the elastic. This can be random – the beauty of the style is that it should look as if you've done it yourself.

4 When all of the hair is secured, lightly apply non-aerosol hairspray.

5 Choose an accessory to suit your outfit.

jet-set hair

Relatively inexpensive air travel has given most of us fast access to the 'global village'. Air travel was once strictly for the jet set, but now that it is no longer exclusive, no one pretends (not even the first-class passengers) that they feel glamorous after a 14-hour flight. Even though the wellbeing programmes on in-flight entertainment give tips on how to exercise (isn't sitting with your knees under your chin exercise?) and avoid dehydration, they never mention how to keep your hair looking as good on arrival as it did on departure.

dehydration

The air pressure in the cabin and the high altitude encourage dehydration, which leaves the skin and hair dull and lacking in radiance. This can only be prevented by drinking copious amounts of water and soft drinks, while avoiding tea, coffee and alcohol, all of which have a diuretic effect that will compound the problem. Drinking carrot and apple juice before a flight will also help to keep hair hydrated.

static

The dry, air-conditioned cabin atmosphere could not be better for static, nor worse for flyaway hair (the wispy rather than the jet-set sort). If you have ever tried brushing or combing your hair while sitting in your seat, you will know that you can hear the crackle of static over the noise of the engines. While there is nothing you can do to change the climate in the cabin, you can counter the static by fixing hair in place with holding wax and gels, which give the hair weight. Resting a headscarf over the headrest will also help to reduce the friction between your hair and the back of the seat.

flaky scalp

Dehydration on board means an increased chance of developing a flaky scalp. If this has happened to you, tie back your hair to avoid dandruff-like flakes on your shoulders. Once you are settled in at your destination, a vigorous but gentle brushing will loosen any flakes.

Follow with a thorough scalp massage to increase the blood flow, and therefore nutrients and oxygen, to the scalp, as well as to release tension from the flight (see page 26). Finally, a shampoo and deep-conditioning treatment will remove any lingering flakes and restore moisture, bounce and shine.

Air-hair dos and don'ts

Don't fly with your hair weighted down with products or your face caked with panstick. Fly with clean hair and a slick of lipstick, if you like.

Do spritz your face regularly with a hydrating mister to keep the skin soft and supple. Use it to refresh stale, dry hair, too.

Do drink plenty of still mineral water.

Don't drink coffee, tea or alcohol.

Do always pack your skincare and haircare products in waterproof bags so there's no chance of them spilling their contents over your favourite silk dress.

Do tie your hair back to help prevent static building up. If you do get static hair, spray some hairspray onto your brush or comb and lightly run it through the hair.

Do pack a gentle, restorative shampoo and super-rich conditioner to revive your travel-stressed hair on arrival.

Do not despair. If you still look less-than-perfect on arrival – despite the litres of water and a first-class seat – simply act like a filmstar and don a pair of dark 'Jackie O' sunglasses, a smart hat, a slick of red lipstick and a disenchanted air.

Never before has the prospect of a business trip to New York seemed quite so exciting as it does now. Apart from the obvious retail opportunities, it's the anticipation of finally meeting cyber-suitor Simon, who has her heart fluttering like a teenager's. There is one problem, though – aeroplane hair – and she has to go straight out from JFK to a dinner meeting uptown with no time for a hotel stop and hair overhaul. After a few hours of being subjected to the two demon hair enemies – static and

... polly's air-hair dilemma

dehydration – Polly's worried that she'll disembark with hair so frizzy and static that the only spark between her and Simon will be the electric shock she gives him when they shake hands for the first time. What to do? Hair in bun? Business-like but maybe too prim. Wear a headscarf? Ladylike-chic but a bit too HRH.

A baseball cap? Very American but not a good look with a suit. Polly hits a brick wall, but a quick phone call to her hair guru, Charles, solves the problem. Drink plenty of H_2O and – top tip – a carrot and apple juice before flying to combat dehydration. Another top tip, put a headscarf on the headrest to prevent static

from the nylon seat covers. Hah! She knew the headscarf would come in handy. Armed with bottles of water and various fruit juice concoctions, her Hermès scarf knotted around her neck, Polly sashays down the corridors at Heathrow's Terminal 4 without a second thought for her boyfriend. Sorry, Harry.

vive la change

We all know someone who has taken the plunge and had the big chop. It usually coincides with a big life change, invariably the end of a relationship. Cutting long hair short is a liberation and, when one considers how men prize long hair, it is a form of emancipation from their – his – ideals. There is bravery attached to a dramatic new look, too. A complete change of colour or a cut – or both – can be tremendously energizing and rejuvenating. Some people thrive on change, whereas others need a gentle nudge to pluck up the courage.

considerations

Whether you're the sort of person who gets a real buzz from reinventing yourself or you take the cautious approach, don't do anything rash. Think carefully about your new look, consider all the options and ask advice from your stylist. The decision to chop off a good four years' growth of hair should not be taken lightly.

1 Think about why you want to have a dramatic change. Remember, a haircut won't bring a lover back or put the world to rights, but it might restore your confidence, perk up your mood and give you a much-needed boost.

2 Are you prepared to change your wardrobe and make-up to accommodate a dramatic new hairstyle? For example, if you are naturally a long-haired brunette, having a short blonde crop will affect the colouring of your face and different clothes will suit you. Be prepared.

3 Copying someone else's style to the letter never works successfully. Find a style or cut that inspires you, then, with the help of your hairstylist, make it your own.

4 A flexible hairstyle is the best one to have. You may love your spiky crop when it's just been done, but get bored with it after the initial impact has worn off.

5 Colour, rather than cut, is the easiest way to effect a big change and yet still leave you with the option to reverse it. A cut is more permanent as it grows out slowly, at little more than 1 cm (½ in) a month.

6 If you are considering cutting long hair, try on a few short-styled wigs beforehand to make sure you like the way it looks on you.

7 If you are thinking of growing out a short haircut, use hairpieces to see if you like the feel of longer hair.

8 Make sure you're ready for a change and don't let anyone push you into doing anything you're not happy about.

9 Think of the upkeep. Will your new look be easy or an effort to style? Will it fit in with your lifestyle? How versatile do you need it to be? And how often will you need to revisit the hairdresser to keep it looking good?

HAIR SNIP

WHEN YOU'RE CONSIDERING GOING FOR A COMPLETE IMAGE-OVERHAUL, LOOK THROUGH LOTS OF BEAUTY AND FASHION MAGAZINES TO FIND AS MANY PICTURES AS YOU CAN OF HAIRSTYLES AND HAIR COLOURS THAT YOU LIKE. TAKE THE WHOLE SELECTION WITH YOU TO THE HAIRDRESSER'S AND YOUR STYLIST WILL HELP YOU DECIDE WHAT ELEMENTS FROM EACH LOOK WILL SUIT YOU AND YOUR HAIR TYPE. THAT WAY, YOU CAN CREATE A UNIQUE LOOK.

gently does it

If you like the idea of changing your image but just can't seem to pluck up the courage to go for a complete reinvention, try a few subtle, temporary changes first. Ask your hairstylist to blow-dry your hair in a different way – if you are naturally curly, get them to blow-dry it dead straight; if you normally wear it forwards, framing your face, ask them to style it away from your face; or have it set in curlers to create gentle waves. If you always wear your hair loose, ask your hairdresser to show you a new way of pinning it up; or simply try parting it in a different way. You could even have a semi-permanent colour rinse that will wash out in a few weeks. All of these devices can make you look and feel quite different without committing yourself to a radical change that will take years to reverse.

If you are flirting with the idea of having short hair, then think about moving up in stages rather than going for a crop in one fell swoop of the scissors. You could evolve from a one-length long cut to a layered Rachel cut, then a shoulder-length bob or a sexy layered 'rock chick' style. You can then try a messed-up Meg Ryan cut and still have hair left to go even shorter. Gradual change is experimental and will give you time to play ideas out and find which styles and cuts suit your face and your personality most.

to fringe or not to fringe?

There are no hard and fast rules about hair type or face shape: some people simply do not suit fringes (bangs). It's a very personal thing. If you are thinking of having a fringe but are not sure if it will suit you, or if you fancy a fringe but don't want anything permanent which you will then have to grow out (a big bore), try faking it. It sounds unlikely but it does work!

How to do it: take a section of hair from the crown, comb it forwards over your forehead and arrange it as you would a fringe. If you've got long hair, twist it to take away the length before taking it forwards. Adjust the width, length and density as required, then clip it securely just above the crown using a large grip. Alternatively, ask your hairstylist to attach a hairpiece. Leave your false fringe for 20 minutes to get used to it before deciding whether it suits you.

moving on

Even the most dramatic changes lose their impact after a time, so the trick is to reinvent your look regularly to avoid getting stuck in a style rut. Think how differently Madonna looks at 40 compared with how she looked in her twenties. Many feel she looks younger now. True to type, she has grown her hair and left it long at the age when most women feel they have to go short. Luckily, hair does grow. So unlike that dolphin tattoo swimming across your buttock, even the most radical change of colour and cut will grow out over time. Be brave and enjoy the positive power of transformation that a radical change can bring. (See overleaf – would you do it?)

without fringe ...

with fringe!

from long . . .

to short!

disco divas party on

Jaz simply could not believe her luck. Squashed up at the bar of Shaft with Laura, while attempting to order yet another round of Cosmopolitans, she'd struck up a conversation with a girl called Imogen, who turned out to be … wait for it … the fashion editor on *Gloss* magazine.

'Sweetie, I love your two-tone hair,' Imogen had declared to Jaz by way of a conversation opener. Jaz, in return, had admired Imogen's fluorescent pink mules, and before she knew it she'd been offered an (unpaid) work placement on *Gloss*. Jaz didn't think twice about accepting. She would quit her job at The Flag on Monday, even if it meant taking an evening job to pay the rent.

In another corner of the crowded bar, Chrissie had Steve the record producer well and truly under her spell – or so she thought. She had been flirting with him relentlessly all evening, purring into his ear and batting her eyelids until she was dizzy. 'Honey, this is a fabulous party … so glad we were able to come along … there are always so many invitations on Saturday nights.' Laura and Jaz listened in to snatches of the conversation, most impressed by Chrissie's small talk, if not by her taste in men.

'OK, Chrissie,' Steve was saying. 'Here's the deal. I'll arrange the interview with Pout. But there's something I want to ask you in return.'
'Yes, honey?' Chrissie flashed him her most winning smile. The audition was in the bag; now he was going to ask her out on a date.
'I was wondering if we could go out to dinner. Sort of a double date – you, me, your flatmate and a friend of mine, John. You see, I really like … Laura.' Laura! Chrissie practically fell off her sky-scraper heels, but thought quickly. Not only was it in the interests of her pop career to go on a double date with Steve, but over three courses and a few bottles of wine she knew she could convince him that it was she, Chrissie, in whom he should be interested. Not boyish, trainer-wearing Laura.
'Oh, I'm sure I can fix up something,' Chrissie purred through gritted teeth.

'No way,' whispered Laura to Jaz. 'He wears leather pants and he looks like a creep. I'm not going on a date with him.' But she hadn't factored in Chrissie's powers of persuasion. By the time the girls left Shaft at 3 am the audition, the double date and a job on *Gloss* were all secured. Result all round – if not exactly what Chrissie had planned.

Across town, poor Kate was swallowing the truly disastrous news that her colour palette should be oyster pinks, peach and … biscuit. Yep, apparently she had to dress in the same shade as a stale digestive in order to get herself noticed at Crunch Biscuits. Life was so unfair; no doubt Prissie Chrissie would be a strawberry-cream or a chocolate-coated cookie.

Meanwhile, on the other side of the pond, Polly's plane was about to touch down at JFK. She hadn't had a wink of sleep – too many glasses of water and trips to the ghastly toilet. And she'd also been too busy feeling guilty about Harry and wondering if cyber-suitor Simon was as sexy as he sounded in his e-mails. Very soon, she would find out.

big date hair

Glamourtime hair is fun – there's nothing like transforming the way you look and feel with a blast of hairspray, a few pins and a bit of styling know-how, and Big Date Hair is the ultimate feel-good experience. It covers your every hair need – whatever the invitation – whether you want to twist up your tresses in a ladylike updo to meet his parents for dinner or gutsy up your mane for a rock chick look that's got to last for as long as you do.

styling basics

the girls catch up

'So it was results all round,' said Chrissie with a self-satisfied smile as she retold the tale of the previous week's party at Shaft, the trendy new bar in Soho. The girls were sitting in Café Marron, their local coffee shop and favourite haunt, filling Polly in on all their news. Or rather, Chrissie was filling her in on their news while the other girls sat sipping their lattes, unable to get a word in edgeways. 'So Jaz got lucky on the job front; Laura was asked out on a date; and I've finally got my audition,' Chrissie recapped triumphantly.

Kate groaned inwardly to herself. Chrissie hadn't stopped banging on about her audition for this stupid new girl band, Pout, all week. Frankly, she was sick of it and it didn't help that she was so bored at work that she was now eating half-pound bags of caramel delights (misshapen and bought at staff discount) daily. It seemed that she, Kate, was destined to spend her days stuck in a dead-end secretarial job, piling on the pounds at Crunch Biscuits, while Chrissie led a fast, glamorous life. She tried to change the subject. 'So, Polly. How was your work trip?' Polly was stirring her cappuccino a little dreamily. 'What? Oh, um, fine, fine,' she said, turning pink and looking a bit flustered. If truth be told, Polly's thoughts were still in the Big Apple rather than in Café Marron. But she couldn't possibly tell the girls about her little moment of passion with Simon, her sexy American colleague. She blushed again as she remembered the long, lingering kiss …

Her flatmates eyed her suspiciously. For someone who had stepped off an overnight flight from New York just a few hours earlier, Polly was looking intriguingly good. Her skin was glowing, her hair looked fashionably dishevelled (as opposed to City-girl neat) and she was wearing stiletto boots with a pair of new, tight, bootleg jeans (bought in SoHo). Polly, sensible Polly, was looking rather foxy 'So did you miss Harry dreadfully?' Kate persisted. 'Harry?' said Polly. 'You know, your boyfriend,' quipped Laura, sarcastically

Fortunately, Polly was saved from answering by Chrissie's burning dilemma. 'I simply can't decide what to wear for my audition,' she was saying. 'It's a toss-up between my lucky red dress – the strapless one – and my snakeskin-print jeans. Jaz, maybe you could style me?' Jaz had been practically bouncing up and down with excitement for the past half hour (and it wasn't the effect of the caffeine). 'Oh, I'd love to. I start my work placement at *Gloss* on Monday, so maybe I'll be able to borrow a designer outfit for you to wear.'

Polly's ears pricked up. 'Work placement? But Jaz, what about your job at The Flag? You do know that a work placement means you don't get paid, don't you?' '*Gloss* is going to pay my travel expenses,' said Jaz, hugging her fuchsia fishnetted knees with excitement. Laura – who had long thought that Jaz came from a completely different planet – stifled a snigger. 'Only travel expenses? How are you going to pay your rent?' asked Polly, dragged back suddenly from her daydream. She was, after all, Jaz's landlady. 'Oh, I'll get an evening job in a bar or something,' said Jaz, her eyes shining at the thought of meeting the world's top fashion designers and models, and travelling across the globe on *Gloss* fashion shoots.

Polly sighed. Life at 23 Havana Road, Shepherds Bush was certainly going to be interesting in the next few weeks. Not least, she thought with a pang of guilt, because sexy Simon had promised to call.

stylist's tool box

You don't need a new haircut or a visit to the salon to achieve wow-factor hair. With a little know-how and the right tools you can perform mini miracles at home. Girls born without curls, for example, can win the battle against nature and give themselves Julia Roberts'-style corkscrews. Similarly, those who are blessed (or cursed, depending on your point of view) with a surfeit of kinks and curls, can make their hair stick-straight, simply by using the right styling products and drying technique. Hair is the ultimate fashion accessory. The golden rule is that if it looks good, you'll feel good. Here's what the professionals have in their tool box:

the gadgets

hairdryer

Not just for blasting wet hair dry, a hairdryer can make your hair sleek and straight, or give it more lift than a pair of Manolos. Make sure yours is at least 1,500 watts, otherwise you will spend valuable date time drying your hair and possibly even damage it in the process.

diffuser

This big, dish-like attachment is used to dry curly hair. It disperses the flow of air so that curls, natural or otherwise, aren't straightened by its sheer force.

brushes

Styling is about shaping the hair, so don't think you can use the same brush as for everyday grooming. Styling brushes come in many shapes and sizes. Flat brushes, which have bristles on one side only, are good, all-round tools, but are not precise enough to curl or straighten the hair. Round brushes, with bristles all the way around, are for curling, straightening or adding volume. Use small-diameter brushes for short hair and large-diameter ones for straightening kinks out of long hair. Broad, flat paddle brushes are great for blow-drying straight or wavy long hair, as well as for styling hair to a poker-straight finish.

combs

You need a good, all-purpose comb for detangling hair, dividing it into sections and for backcombing.

curling tongs

These create curls for girls who don't have them. Use small-diameter tongs for short hair or for making tight curls, and large tongs for creating looser curls in long hair. You can also get heated curling brushes, which have bristles rather than a clamp to hold the hair in place. Use tongs on dry hair only.

straightening irons

These are used after blow-drying to give a blunt, poker straight look. The two flat, heated plates are clamped over a section of hair and slowly drawn down to the ends. They should not be used too often as they are very dehydrating.

crimping irons

As well as creating the distinctive 'corrugated' wave that goes in and out of fashion faster than flared trousers, these irons can also be used on the under layers of dry hair to boost volume, or at the roots to lift limp hair.

rollers

Rollers, which can be used to add volume to hair as well as make it curly, have become very hip. And hurrah for the fact that – unlike your grandmother's generation – you don't have to go to bed wearing them. Heated rollers (for use on dry hair only) are a speedy way of creating strong curls. For loose curls, take out the rollers while they are still warm. Velcro rollers are non-heated but you can put them into dry or damp hair to add lift at the roots.

hairpins, grips and sectioning clips

Small hairpins and grips are essential for securing updos and small sections of hair – use matt ones, which are less slippery, in a colour that matches your hair. Big metal clips are useful when you need to hold larger sections of hair up and out of the way for styling.

Chrissie is leaving nothing to chance. Tomorrow is her big audition with Pout, so she's locked herself in the bathroom for yet another experiment. She knows it's going to annoy Kate, who's already started to make snide comments about Chrissie hogging the bathroom all the time, but it just can't be helped. Chrissie's determined to turn her fine blonde hair into big hair and the way to do it, she's read in one of her many beauty books, is to use extra-large rollers. Standing in front of the bathroom mirror, she finishes rolling the last big Velcro roller snugly

... chrissie tries big hair for size

against her scalp (for maximum volume) and spritzes her hair with styling spray. Ten minutes later Chrissie carefully removes the rollers and admires herself with a satisfied (almost smug – Laura would call it narcissistic) smile. Not only does her hair look bigger and bouncier, but the strapless red dress shows off her fake tan to perfection. Jaz has tried to convince her to wear her python-print jeans and a pussy-cat bow blouse, but Chrissie knows better. The other girls from Pout practically live in snakeskin-print jeans, and she wants to look different. In her tight scarlet dress (holding her hairbrush to her mouth in mock singing/karaoke mode) and with her limp blonde locks transformed into big voluminous hair, there is no doubt that Chrissie is going to stand out from the crowd ...

the products

If you don't know a serum from a shine spray, the range of styling lotions and potions out there is enough to make your hair curl. But you don't need a whole battery of products: the contents of your personal tool box will depend on your particular hair type and the style that you want to achieve.

wax and pomade

Wax and pomade are designed to add definition and hold. They come in numerous strengths, holds and consistencies, so it might take a while to find the best one for you – but once you've found it, you won't ever want to be without it.

anti-frizz serum

This is the product for eliminating frizzy, flyaway bits and for bringing unruly hair to heel. It contains silicone, which coats the hair shaft and smooths and seals the cuticle. Use it on wet hair before styling or to smooth down dry hair. Serum can be mixed with other products to give extra-glossy drying and extra protection.

curl revitalizer and activator

These perk up deflated curls by adding moisture – but only if the curl existed in the first place. These products tend to come in gel form, and the more product used, the more defined the curl. Test these products before a big night out, as too much can sometimes overload the hair.

styling crème

Similar to leave-in conditioner, this acts as a form of damage limitation if you apply it to the ends of the hair before using heated appliances. Volume control or non-chemical relaxers normally come in a cream form and should be used sparingly.

shine enhancer

This usually comes in spray or liquid form and contains silicone to coat the hair shaft, smooth the cuticle and add the magic shine factor. Shine spray is an absolute must-have for perfect, glossy, glamour hair.

mousse

A light and airy foam that is used to add oomph to fine hair (apply it to the roots before blow-drying) or to shape and control dry hair. Mousse comes in varying strengths and can be used for softer setting techniques.

volumizer and thickener

These pump up the volume on pancake-flat or very fine hair by swelling the hair shaft. They work best when applied near the roots before blow-drying. They tend not to overload the hair, since they are designed for fine hair. So, for more volume and hold, use more product.

gel

Gel can be used to slick back unruly hair, giving good hold and a glossy finish. Light-hold gels may also be used in curly hair to define the curls, or in fine hair to give volume.

hairspray

The original styling product, this is still used after styling to hold hair in place. Useful for updos and styles that need to keep their shape. Hairsprays come in different strengths, so choose one for your desired hold. Hairspray also helps to reduce static.

back to basics

Before you start transforming your tresses with rollers, plaits and updos, master the fundamental styling techniques for best results. For great curls see page 60 and for super-sleek straight hair see page 63.

big hair

you need
Hairdryer • volumizing mousse or blow-drying spray • sectioning clips • brush with a detachable bristle roller • hairspray

1 After shampooing and conditioning, blow-dry the hair roughly until it is 70 per cent dry.

2 Apply the mousse or blow-drying spray, working it evenly through the hair with your fingers.

3 Pin up the top layer of the hair with sectioning clips so that you can access the layer underneath. Dry the hair section by section, using the roller brush to hold the roots at right angles to the scalp as you do so to give maximum volume.

4 Unclip the top layer section by section and dry each one in the same way, this time unclipping the handle of the brush and leaving the roller in the hair to set in volume. This creates a soft fullness that lifts the hair away from the head. It also smooths and softens the hair cuticles, maximizing gloss and shine.

5 Give the hair a blast of cold air to set, then gently remove the brush head once the hair is completely cool.

6 When you have finished drying all the hair, shape it with your fingers and lightly spritz with hairspray.

textured hair

you need
Medium-hold gel • comb • hairdryer

1 A quick, easy way of adding texture to hair of any length is to apply a little medium-hold gel to the root area. You can do this on wet hair or dry hair.

2 Using a hairdryer, direct the heat at the roots and use your fingers to lift the hair as you do so.

3 Once the roots are dry, take the heat through to the ends of your hair, combing it with your fingers. This gives a slightly messy and windblown look.

4 For ultimate 'rock chick' texture and great volume, finish by tipping your head upside-down and gently roughing up the hair with your hands.

styling secrets

Always finish blow-drying your hair with a quick blast of cold air. Not only does it 'set' the new shape in place, but it closes the hair cuticles which maximizes gloss and shine. (When the cuticles lie flat, they reflect the light better.) Now that's a cute tip!

For best blow-drying results, gently dry the hair until it is 70 per cent dry before attempting to style it – trying to style and shape wet hair is just a waste of time and effort.

Be careful when you dry your hair upside-down – it can rough up the cuticle which leaves the hair looking dull. Only do it occasionally if you want to build up huge volume.

When using waxes and serums, the secret is to start off with a tiny amount and add more gradually if it is needed.

Always use a clean hairbrush – not one that is clogged up with hair and product. You should wash your brushes once a week in a little shampoo and warm water.

'It must be the effect of living with looks-obsessed Chrissie and Jaz,' thinks Laura as she towel-dries her hair at the gym and contemplates making her gamine crop ... well, a little more interesting. Laura normally relishes the fact that she can jump out of the shower, blast her short hair dry and pull on her combats and trainers – all within ten minutes of finishing her kick-boxing class. Tonight, however, she has half an hour

... laura glams up her gamine crop

to kill before setting off for an important work party. 'Well, I might as well give it a go,' thinks Laura as she reaches into her gym bag for the little pot of styling wax that Chrissie gave her the night before. 'It'll gutsy-up your hair,' Chrissie had said – whatever that meant. Laura

usually has little time for Chrissie and her unsolicited beauty tips, but she wants to make an effort tonight. She works the wax into the ends as Chrissie had instructed, then blasts them dry, using her fingertips for lift. By the time she's finished, her hair looks sexy and tousled – as though

she's just climbed out of bed. Laura's impressed (in a rather understated, Laura kind of way). John, the devastatingly attractive assistant producer from Current Affairs, is likely to be at the party – and Laura's more than ready for a spot of networking – if that's what you want to call it.

colour me beautiful

Adding a touch of colour, whether it is permanent, semi-permanent or temporary, is a great way to perk up hair that is looking dull and lifeless, and a brilliant way to change your look or revolutionize your style. If the words 'shrinking' and 'violet' could never be used in the same sentence to describe you, then try adding a shock of bright colour – this adds punch to any hairstyle. The more faint-hearted can either boost and enhance their natural hair colour or get a little adventurous with some creative colour. How about a few strands of a contrasting shade around your face, for example? Or, what about getting just the very tips of your hair dipped in a daring bright colour? Either way, don't be afraid of colour; it can be really fun and opens up loads of opportunities for transforming yourself – à la Madonna, the mistress of reinvention.

something for the weekend?

The great thing about temporary colour is that it's, well ... temporary. It provides the perfect opportunity for trying out something new or for making an impact without causing any long-lasting and irreversible consequences. There'll be no crying over spilt milk with temporary colour!

It is always a good idea to pick your hairdresser's brains about colour before you launch yourself into the rainbow of choices and techniques available. Find out what colours they think will suit your skin tone and what formulations and techniques will have the best effect and results on your hair type.

colour wash

This easy wash-in, wash-out colour rinse lasts for just one shampoo and is good for subtle shade enhancement. Colour washes are also known as vegetable colours and are excellent for refreshing faded colour and conditioning the hair.

semi-permanent colour rinse

This is a vegetable-based dye that lasts for up to approximately 12 shampoos. You can only go darker or warmer than your natural colour.

coloured spray

As well as adding oomph to simpler styles, such as plaits, this can be used to create an all-over effect. You could, for example, spray hair in a mist of silver to match a silver party dress – Barbarella, eat your heart out!

colour mousse

This is good for toning down brassiness or changing your colour for the night. It is best to seek professional advice as some leave a coloured 'cast' on the hair.

wax and pomade

These are applied after the hair has been dried and styled. It's always advisable to do a test strand with stronger colours to make sure it doesn't stain the hair and will wash out – especially if you have blonde or bleached hair. This product is best used on small areas.

hair mascara

The wand makes it really easy to streak colour through your hair. Use it around the front section of your hair and on the strands framing your face for best results. Be warned: test out hair mascaras at the beauty counter first as a colour that looks pretty in a tube can look pretty dull (or unnoticeable) on your hair.

creative colour

Creative colour, as it's known in the salon, tends to be semi-permanent or permanent, so it's a great choice if you're feeling funky and want a look that's going to last longer than a couple of washes. As its name suggests, creative colour is where a hairstylist gets creative and even more artistic – your hair is a canvas on which colour application and technique converge. Some creative-colour techniques can produce quite radical results, so talk it through with your hairdresser and make sure you know exactly what you're letting yourself in for. Your gorgeous tie-dye locks may not be appreciated if you work in a bank or law firm!

If you're longing to try techniques like dip-dyeing or tie-dyeing but think they sound a bit radical and long-lasting, you can cheat by colouring hairpieces and then weaving them into your hair.

dip-dyeing
This technique (left), inspired by the art of dip-dyeing clothes, is where just the very ends of your hair are coloured. It works best on natural, mid-length to long hair and you can use either subtle or vibrant colours. For the most dramatic results, have your ends dip-dyed in a contrasting colour to your natural shade. For example, if your hair is dark brown or black, dip-dye the ends pillar-box red.

couture colour
Your hair is shaded with colour to personalize and complement your haircut, making it unique to you. This type of colour enhances movement and emphasizes a dramatic line.

tonal blast
This is a more subtle version of dip-dyeing that works best on short to mid-length textured haircuts. The ends of the hair are coloured and then a semi-permanent colour wash is applied over the top to give extra brightness and a strong tone of colour. A tonal blast can be done on all natural or coloured hair, with the exception of hair that has already been dyed black.

3-D lights
Slices of hair are coloured with shades of blonde all over the head; darker blonde is applied at the roots and lighter blonde to the ends to give a sun-kissed look. This works best on short to mid-length hair and can be done on all shades of natural or coloured blonde hair.

hidden colour
Sections of hair are taken from underneath and coloured, which makes 'work-to-play' hair easy – clip up your hair to reveal the drama below. This works best on all natural hair colours and on mid-length to long hair.

duo colour
The hair is either coloured lighter on top and darker underneath or darker on top and lighter underneath. This can be done on all natural or coloured hair and works best on mid-length to long hair. Trio colour involves using three contrasting colours.

hang loose

spoiling themselves at the spa

Wrapped in fluffy white robes, the girls sat clutching cups of calming herbal tea while having their toes pedicured in the calm cream reception area of their favourite spa. Their faces were as long as Chrissie's newly-painted acrylic nails. It had not been a good week, so they had decided to cheer themselves up with a little bit of pampering. Good old Polly had even offered to pay for Jaz, who could not have afforded to go otherwise. The soothing tinkle of the feng-shui water wall and the prospect of a massage with hot stones (the latest beauty treatment) had already helped to lift their spirits.

'Poor Jaz,' thought Polly. Her dream work placement on *Gloss* magazine had not turned out to be quite as glamorous as she had expected. For the past week she had been incarcerated in the windowless fashion cupboard, sorting out the tights and set free only to fetch organic wheatgrass juice for Imogen, the fashion editor. As for meeting a fashion designer, she was about as likely to meet Elvis.

'Pass me that copy of The Rainbow, please Jaz. I need to work on my new image,' barked Chrissie. She had become even more obsessed with her looks since Pout had proclaimed her 'too womanly' to join their band. She was devastated about it but, in true Chrissie style, only for about two seconds. Instead, she had accepted the job of receptionist at Devastation Records that Steve had offered her by way of compensation. He had hinted that if she took the job, there was a chance that she might be 'discovered'. 'Too right I will,' Chrissie had thought, resolving there and then to be the most glamorous (and girliest) receptionist ever. 'And to think I wore my lucky red dress,' she thought aloud to herself, while admiring her newly-painted, mink-coloured toenails (the perfect accompaniment to her long, honey-coloured calves, she thought). 'Yes, but look at what you wore with the red dress,'

pointed out Laura, characteristically as blunt as the cut of her boyish crop. 'Those turquoise tights that Jaz persuaded you to wear looked ridiculous!'

'Laura, don't be mean to Chrissie,' said Polly looking up from the work file she had brought along with her for light reading – anything to take her mind off the fact that Simon had not called. Worse still, his once-flirtatious e-mails had become very brisk and matter-of-fact. And to top it all, Polly was feeling really guilty about Harry, who seemed to have finally woken up to her existence. He had actually paid her a compliment about her new 'messy' hair (as he called it) and had even presented her with a bunch of flowers – even though they were carnations.

'I think I might go for the slimming seaweed wrap,' declared Kate, who had been scanning the menu of beauty treatments. Out of all the girls, Kate secretly had something to celebrate. She had managed to lose a bit of weight since switching to a new, low-fat brand of biscuit that was being trial-tested at Crunch. Matthew was currently racking his brains, trying to think of a name for them. Kate, however, had already thought of one. It was time to convince her gorgeous boss that her talents stretched to more than just typing letters and doing the filing.

Laura was also studying the treatments on offer. Beauty spas were not usually her thing, but she had willingly agreed when Polly suggested it. She had to do something to get John's attention. At the TV party where she had planned to 'bump' into him, he had spent the entire time talking to a girl with long, curly hair who was wearing a flowery frock. 'Chrissie's worried about looking too womanly, but maybe my problem,' thought Laura, as she helped herself to an apple, 'is that I'm not womanly enough. Still, it was never too late for a cynical 26-year-old TV researcher to learn a beauty trick or two.

straight talking

Straight is not as straightforward as you might think. You can take your pick from straight and dishevelled, straight and sleek or straight with lots of volume. There are as many ways to wear your hair loose as there are shades of lipstick. Hair worn down is a great seduction tool: you can indulge in flirtatious ploys, like tossing it back or running your fingers through it (although strictly speaking, this is a no-no as it can make hair look greasy). That said, the secret to great date hair is a style that somebody else wants to run their fingers through ...

big straight hair

Big straight hair is all about boosting thickness without weighing down the hair. Here's the lowdown:

you need
Wide flat brush (ideally a paddle brush) • hairdryer • crimping irons • straightening irons • sectioning clips • non-aerosol hairspray

1 Follow the instructions on page 63 for blow-drying and straightening your hair with straightening irons.

2 Pin the top layers of your hair out of the way, using the sectioning clips.

3 Take the underneath layers, section by section, and lightly spritz the root area with hairspray to protect it from the heat of the crimping iron, then crimp the hair close to the roots.

4 When you have crimped the roots of all the underneath layers, gently comb the crimped sections out and then let the hair you have pinned away fall over the top.

Spurred on by her weight loss (it was a good start) and her indulgent day at the spa (she definitely felt more toned after the seaweed wrap), Kate decides that Sunday night is going to be

... kate's power bob goes straight

'an achieve salon-style hair at home' night. She furtively eyes the carrier bag that contains her latest purchase. It's over a month since she walked into her hairdresser's and demanded a power bob. What she had been given – a shoulder-length bob-shaped cut – was as close to a power bob as you can get when you possess flowing, unruly titian locks. But Kate hankers after bone-straight hair – the mark of the sleek, sophisticated

career babe. She is positive that with the right hair she could get ahead in the Crunch marketing department. Like a woman with a serious mission, she plugs in her new straightening irons to let them heat up while she sections off her hair as instructed by the accompanying booklet. She can hardly believe the transformation that takes place as she carefully runs the irons down each section. In less than half an hour she goes from

pre-Raphaelite maiden to a smart, take-me-seriously hotshot. She knows that she can't do this sort of thing too often (overuse of straightening irons being very damaging to the hair), but once in a while can't possibly hurt. Delighted with her new image (she even looks as sharp and business-like as Polly), she decides that tomorrow is the day to broach the subject of accompanying Matthew on that important conference.

blades

There's straight, there's big straight and then there's 'Gucci-style' straight, which leaves your hair looking like blades of grass all over. (Hence the salon-speak for this look is simply 'blades'.) It's a very sharp look that makes your hair seem almost crispy. But be warned: this technique involves hot straightening irons and is potentially dehydrating to the hair if used regularly, so it is best saved for big dates only.

you need

hairdryer • straightening brush • pump-action hairspray • straightening irons

1 Follow the instructions on page 63 for blow-drying your hair straight.

2 Using a pump-action rather than an aerosol hairspray, spritz the hair until it is quite damp. (A pump-action hairspray releases a higher volume of product, which makes the hair damper.) Do this evenly down the entire length of your hair.

3 Take a small 2.5-cm (1-inch) wide section of hair and slowly run the straightening irons down it, from the roots to the ends.

4 Repeat this process all over the head, being sure to straighten the underneath layers and not just the top section. This should leave the hair totally separated into small individual 'blades'.

bed-head hair

There is something very sexy about slightly dishevelled or shaggy hair, also known as 'bed-head hair' because it looks like you've just climbed out of bed and not bothered to brush it. On long hair, this look is also labelled 'Rock Chick' – messy, but sexy, as sported by Chrissie Hynde, Courtney Love and Marianne Faithful.

you need

Light-hold mousse or gel spray • hairdryer • paddle brush • hairspray

1 Apply a little mousse or gel spray to the root area of the hair using your fingers to work it through.

2 Rough-dry the hair. Instead of sectioning off the hair and blow-drying each piece separately, randomly blast the hair with the hairdryer, gently roughing it up with your fingers. This will maximize the volume and give a really shaggy finish.

3 Lightly spritz with hairspray to hold the look.

short and spiky

Don't think that just because you've got short hair you have limited styling options. There's a lot you can do with short hair – you can make it soft, sexy and tousled; slick it back neatly for understated glossy elegance; decorate it with pretty hair slides and grips; or spike it up for a groovy, street-chick look – all you need is a range of good styling products, some basic tools and a little bit of know-how. This funky textured look (right) is a great way to make short hair more gutsy, and will certainly get you noticed.

you need

Strong-hold gel • hairspray • hairdryer and diffuser

1 Apply a generous amount of strong-hold gel to wet hair, using your fingers to distribute the product evenly to the ends and gently work the hair into spikes.

2 Dry your hair with your head tipped over, using a diffuser to help keep all of the spikes intact.

3 Finally, spray your hair with hairspray to add extra hold and shine.

plait it, braid it

laits are not just for schoolgirls – they can look very elegant, very hip or very sexy. There are loads of variations – from a single braid hanging straight down your back to a whole headful of braiding finished with beads. If you don't want all of your hair in a plait, just braid a small section of the hair anywhere you like to add extra texture and interest. The most popular way to do this is to plait a small section on either side of the face and then take these around the side of the head and clip them at the back. Very Guinevere!

the multiplait

This is a very beautiful, very simple style of wearing your hair down your back in a neat, elegant, textural plait.

you need

Comb • sectioning clips • three covered elastic bands • hairspray or anti-frizz serum

HAIR SNIP
TO AVOID HAVING A BIG CHUNKY BAND AT THE END OF YOUR PLAIT. FINISH IT OFF BY LIGHTLY BACKCOMBING THE TIPS OF THE HAIR. ALTERNATIVELY, USE CLEAR, SNAG-FREE ELASTIC BANDS FOR LARGER PLAITS OR BEADS FOR SMALLER PLAITS.

FRENCH PLAITS WILL LOOK NEATER AND STAY TIGHTER FOR LONGER IF YOU ADD IN VERY SMALL SECTIONS OF HAIR AT EACH TURN. ALWAYS PLAIT THEM TIGHT AGAINST THE SCALP.

FOR A PLAIT WITH A DIFFERENCE, WEAVE IN COLOURFUL RIBBONS OR STRIPS OF LEATHER, YOU CAN ALSO DECORATE PLAITS WITH FLOWERS AND FEATHERS.

1 Divide your hair into three sections: one on the left, one at the back and one on the right.

2 Divide the left section into three, plait it near the nape and secure it with a hair band.

3 Plait the right section in the same way, leaving the middle section unplaited.

4 Then plait all three sections together for an interesting combination of textures.

5 Finally, use hairspray or an anti-frizz serum to flatten any stray hairs.

sexy plaits

These are sexy, bad-girl plaits!

you need

Comb • sectioning clips • three snag-free elastic bands • shine spray • straightening irons

1 Divide the hair into three sections from the front of the head to the nape, leaving out a small section at the front to flop seductively over one eye.

2 French-plait the first section tightly onto the scalp, following the shape of the head. This is important as it will ensure that the plait is tight towards the nape.

3 Leave about 15 cm (6 in) unplaited at the end. Fold this back and secure it with a snag-free elastic.

4 Repeat with the other two plaits, then spritz the hair with shine spray (see opposite).

5 Finish by straightening the loose front section.

girls with curls

the same way as girls with the most beautiful curly
locks at times lust after flat-ironed hair, those born
with naturally straight tresses long for a cascade of
tumbling curls. Maybe it's because the grass is always
greener ... Straightening or curling, you can't defy
nature permanently, but you can have a lot of fun.

Curls come in many different guises: from the softest
Madonna-style wave to tight corkscrews and romantic
Jane Austen ringlets. Even if your hair is naturally
as straight as a ruler, it's easy to create the curls of
your dreams at home.

wavy hair

The best way to achieve long-lasting, glossy curls is
to use curling tongs. It is important to work on freshly
washed hair (too much product on the hair will make
look dull when you use tongs).

you need
Comb • hairspray • curling tongs • glossing spray

1 Starting at the nape of the neck, divide the hair
into quite chunky sections (about 9 cm/3½ in wide).

2 Lightly spray the first section with
hairspray to ensure a longer-lasting curl.

3 Comb it through to remove any product build-up
before clamping the tongs over the ends of the
section, making sure they are completely tucked in.

4 Gently wind the tongs up, making sure
that all the hair is covering the metal barrel.
Hold for about 4–10 seconds, depending on
the heat of the tongs and the curl required,
then gently unwind. (Be careful not to run
your fingers through the curled section.)

5 Repeat this process until all of your hair has
been tonged, then lightly spray it with a light
glossing spray to finish.

ringlets

If you have naturally curly hair, creating ringlets is easy.
This technique is also a good way to avoid frizzy curls.

you need
Serum • styling gel • comb • finishing spray

1 Simply rub serum and gel together in the palm
of one hand. Apply to wet hair and comb it through.

2 Leave your hair to dry naturally and the
hair will form ringlets. For a bit of extra help,
take sections of hair and twist them around
your finger before leaving to dry.

3 For a glossy finish, lightly spritz with finishing spray.

If you have straight hair, there are several methods
of creating ringlets. The old-fashioned technique of
'ragging', using torn-up bits of cloth (strips of J-cloth
works especially well), has made a twenty-first
century comeback. Once mastered, it is quicker and
better than using rollers.

you need
Medium-hold styling spray • strips of cloth •
hairdryer and diffuser (optional)

1 Start by spritzing the hair with medium-hold styling
spray (use quite a lot to give a firm, springy curl).

2 Beginning at the nape of the neck, divide
the hair into sections depending on the size
of ringlet required. (Continued on page 118.)

3 Wrap the hair around the cloth, being careful to tuck in the ends neatly. For a more defined ringlet, slightly twist each section as you wind it up.

4 Once the hair is wound tightly around the strip of cloth, snug to the scalp, tie the two ends of the cloth together.

5 When all the hair is tied, either leave it to dry naturally (the rags are comfortable enough to sleep in), or use a hairdryer and diffuser – but this can be time-consuming.

6 When you are sure that the hair is dry, start to remove the rags, beginning at the nape of the neck.

7 When all the rags have been removed, use your fingers to gently break up the curls, depending on how curly or defined you want the final effect.

afro-style

You don't even need to have curly hair to create a cloud of tight Afro curls. Even poker-straight tresses can be transformed to get this effect.

you need
Strong setting lotion • strips of silver foil • wide-tooth comb

1 Spritz the hair thoroughly with strong setting lotion to give a more defined curl.

2 Follow the instructions for ragging (see above), but take much smaller sections of hair and instead of winding the hair around strips of cloth, use small pieces of foil.

3 When you remove the pieces of foil, instead of running your fingers through the hair, use a wide-tooth comb. This will totally separate the curls, leaving you with a perfect Afro.

big curls

you're not satisfied with Madonna-style waves or a
eadful of ringlets, then big curls (with a capital B) are
e order of the day. Reach out for the hot rollers for
bit of va-va-voom.

ou need
lousse • hairdryer • hairspray • heated rollers

To create the perfect foundation for a hot-roller
et, apply mousse to the root area of freshly
ashed hair. Then, using the warm setting on
our hairdryer, dry the mousse into the hair.

2 Take a section of hair, making sure it's
not wider than the actual roller, and spray
it evenly with hairspray.

3 Wind the section around the end of the first
ller, tucking in the ends. Make sure that the roller
ts firmly against the scalp as this will create root
t and a much bouncier curl.

4 When you've finished putting all of
the hair in rollers, apply a coat of hairspray
evenly all over. Leave the rollers in for about
10 minutes before gently unrolling them.
Don't tug or pull the rollers out.

AIR SNIP

IAKE SURE THAT THE ENDS OF THE HAIR ARE
UCKED IN WHEN YOU CURL THE HAIR AROUND
HE ROLLERS, TONGS OR RAGS, OTHERWISE YOU
ILL END UP WITH A FISH-HOOK EFFECT AT THE
ND OF THE CURL.

AIT FOR THE HOT ROLLERS TO GO COLD
EFORE REMOVING THEM AS THIS WILL CLOSE
HE CUTICLES OF THE HAIR AND SET THE CURLS.

PRAY EACH SECTION WITH SHINE SPRAY AS YOU
EMOVE THE ROLLER TO GUARANTEE GLOSSY
ND VOLUMINOUS CURLS.

Jaz is dreading the prospect of another boring afternoon in the fashion cupboard, bagging up clothes from the glamorous shoots that she never gets to go on. Imogen announces that she's simply going have to go home with another one of her stress headaches (although Jaz can't see exactly what stress her boss is under since all she does is chat on the phone all day to her friends, dahling). She wonders, would Jaz mind going to the launch of Blast, Jean-Paul's new perfume, after work in her place? Jaz would just about manage … Stifling a squeal, she tries to look nonchalant, but not very effectively. Anyway, the coast is now clear for the rest of the afternoon and she has a party to get ready for. Jaz has been dying to try on that amazing purple dress from Coletta, and perhaps a new hairstyle would be just the thing to cheer her up. Emboldened, she manages to get herself an appointment with *Gloss*'s favoured hairstylist, Adam, and begs him to create something awesome for the launch that night. He patiently crimps every bit of her long, dark glossy hair, backcombing

… jaz goes crazy with the crimpers

it at the roots for extra volume. 'Hmm, not bad,' thinks Jaz. Flicking through a back issue of *Gloss*, she spots a great photograph of a catwalk model with plaits wrapped around the side of her head. Adam obligingly braids the front sections of her hair into four small plaits, tying the ends with coloured ribbon. The effect is Kate Bush meets Guinevere – altogether quite pleasing. Jaz is thrilled. Falling off her precarious pin stiletto heels, she rushes out of the salon towards her oh-so-chic destination, but not before giving Adam a massive hug in gratitude. 'I'll do you a favour,' she shrieks, almost tripping up as she tries to hail a cab. 'I won't hold my breath,' thinks Adam, 'but she is a real cutie.'

glamourtime tips

1 Accessorize, accessorize, accessorize. There are so many clever, simple accessories on the market that can be used to make an instant change from dawn to night.

2 Glam up any style by using a sparkle gel or spray glitter along your parting.

3 If you are going to a hot, sweaty party, backcomb the hair at the root to keep the hair big all night.

4 Outshine any rivals: to polish the hair and make it super-shiny, rub a few drops of serum into the palm of your hand, then sweep a large make-up brush across your hand and smooth it down the hair shaft. This is especially effective on long hair.

5 Apply coloured hair mascara – in gold, copper, blonde or a shade lighter than your own – to strands around your face for instant do-it-yourself highlights.

6 Scent your hair by spraying a cloud of perfume into the air and then walking through it. Hair holds perfume really well, so this seductive little trick should create wafts of gorgeousness every time you flick your hair or turn your head.

7 Hold your hair away from your face with beautiful jewelled clips, or pin it back with a big fake flower.

8 For a super-quick, super-dramatic solution, use a ponytail extension (see page 144).

9 Gently curl the ends of ruler-straight hair using tongs to create contrasting texture.

10 Randomly crimp sections of your hair to create volume and a multitextured look.

11 Twist curly sections into full bundles and secure them with glitzy hair grips.

12 Jazz up poker-straight hair by randomly plaiting sections throughout, even plaiting coloured ribbon into them.

13 If you're working the party circuit and styling your hair a lot, you may find that your hair becomes heavy and lank due to a build-up of products. Simply use a detoxifying shampoo for a thorough cleanse.

14 Experiment with a wig – why not be someone else for a night?

15 Overuse of heated styling appliances can damage or dry the hair, so always make sure that you follow instructions carefully. If you are concerned that your hair is becoming dry, use a rich, conditioning hair treatment or mask once a week to replenish moisture.

16 To give your naturally straight hair a bit of texture, plait damp hair before you go to bed. When you wake up, apply a little serum to your fingertips and run them through the hair to undo the plaits. Or, for a quick fix, apply hairspray to dry hair and plait it. Leave it for half an hour and then undo the plaits to get crinkley waves.

17 When choosing your parting, look at what you're wearing. Pick out a feature like the shape of your neckline and follow this when styling your parting.

hair dressing

Hair accessories, like fringes (bangs), are a very personal thing. Some might love a big fake lily poking out from behind the ear; others may not. Hair slides, clips, feathers, flowers and all sorts of glittery bits and bobs can make a great finishing flourish, but they go in and out of fashion faster than you can say 'Kirby grip', so don't waste money on expensive pieces, and be sure to play around with them first before buying them.

tiaras and headbands

Tiaras can look great with long or short hair, but the trick is to wear them with irony (think Courtney Love rather than royalty). We can thank fashion gurus for the revival of headscarves and bandanas. A brightly patterned scarf worn bandana-style over long, straight hair can look very cool. (It's also a great way to cover up on a bad-hair day!)

Head bands come in a range of widths, materials and finishes, whether you want to opt for a minimal strip of leather or a kitsch band with beaded flowers attached to the side. Make sure they fit properly and comfortably.

do-it-yourself accessories

It's amazing what you can make in the way of hair accessories using old pieces of jewellery. You can wire brooches onto combs; glue beads or sequins onto slides; or thread beads onto wire and attach them to hair grips. You can even use a diamanté necklace or bracelet to decorate your hair – simply drape it over your hair and secure it in place with a few matt hair grips.

Glue decorative coloured feathers onto thin strips of leather – either natural or dyed a bright colour – and then attach them to matt hair grips.

Wrap fine florist's wire around the stems of fresh flowers, individually or arranged in small posies, and attach them to hair slides, grips or combs.

clips

Beautiful glittery, jewelled, beaded or feathered clips are one of the best and easiest forms of hair ornament. They can either be attached randomly throughout the hair or placed at the side to keep hair back from the face.

flowers

A big flower – real or fake – pinned behind the ear or at the back of the head is a great way to 'dress up' not only your hair, but also a simple outfit for a big date.

glitter sprays and gels

You only have to look at the big trend for iridescent and glittery face and body make-up to realize that sparkle and shine are definitely 'in'. Try adding a bit of glitter to strands of hair around the face to brighten up your complexion and put you in the party mood.

great lengths

If you want to hang loose but your hair doesn't even reach your jaw line, don't despair. You don't have to wait for your hair to grow, you can get a head start by faking it with hairpieces, extensions and wigs. No longer the domain of the follically challenged, these hairpieces are amazingly realistic, and, more to the point, they allow you to experiment with looks you could otherwise never achieve. Sport a sexy, gamine crop by day and a Rapunzel-like mane by night!

faking it

Clip-on extensions and hairpieces are a great way to add volume or length to your hair. But in order to weave some practical magic with a hairpiece, you do need to have a bit of length already, as they look better when they blend with existing hair (see page 144 for instructions on how to attach them).

To achieve 'extreme long hair', attach five to ten narrow 60-cm (23½-in) hairpieces from the nape to the crown of the head using toupee clips. These are slightly rounded so they sit nice and flat on the head. If your hair is shorter, you could try fake ponytails or plaits, which are attached with clips or combs.

wig tips

1 To make a wig look more natural, have it cut on your head by your hairdresser (razor-cutting techniques tend to work and look best).

2 To give a wig extra body and to make it look less fake, try crimping the roots.

3 If you have a long, straight wig in a colour that is a close match to your own hair, a great trick is to cut small sections out of it and pull strands of your own hair through it. Blending the wig with your own hair in this way not only makes the wig look more convincing, but also prevents it from slipping off your head.

4 If you are wearing a wig over long hair and want it to sit more closely to the scalp, cover your head with the foot of a popsock and put the wig on over the top.

5 When washing wigs or hairpieces, always seek professional advice; not all wigs are made from human hair and they may need special care and attention.

6 Be very careful when you handle wigs and hairpieces – they are woven onto a weft so they are very delicate.

7 Ask to see the actual wig or hairpiece you wish to buy, as natural hairpieces are different in colour and may vary from the colour chart.

emergency quick fixes

1 To revive or add volume to hair when there is no time to wash it, simply spritz the roots with blow-drying spray and then dry the hair, focusing on the root area.

2 If your hair starts to droop, tip your head upside down and spritz the roots with hairspray. Don't be tempted to put too much product on the ends of the hair as it will just drag it down.

3 A handy trick: if your hair has collapsed from too much energetic dancing in a club, or if you don't have access to a blow-dryer, spritz the roots with hairspray and use the hand-dryer in the cloakroom to dry it.

4 When you are pinning up your hair with hair grips, lightly backcomb the roots as this will give a longer-lasting hold.

5 If all else fails, tie your hair back in a low ponytail, securing it at the nape. For an extra-tight hold, wrap it with a piece of wet string instead of a hair band – the string will contract as it dries.

SOS tool kit

Make space for the following in your bag and you need never have another bad-hair moment again!

comb or brush
This one goes without saying.

covered elastic band
With one of these you can always pull your hair back in an emergency.

multifunction styling spray
Use this for holding updos in place or giving an emergency lift to hair that's looking a little limp.

five matt hair grips
These will enable you to fix your hair in a sleek chignon or updo and go straight out from work to play. Matt hair grips don't slip out of the hair and don't show as much as shiny ones.

serum
This silicone-based wonder product will smooth out any frizz and give a sleek, shiny finish.

updos

a quiet night in washing hair

'The pizzas have arrived,' yelled Polly, entering the kitchen with a stack of boxes. It was Thursday and the girls were having a quiet night in washing their hair. Things were looking up for all of them. Chrissie had finally cajoled Laura into going on that double date – drinks and dinner in the Rush bar tomorrow. Meanwhile, Kate's boss had asked her to attend the biscuit conference in Birmingham. This – she couldn't believe her luck – was to be followed by a gala dinner. 'OK, so it's not exactly a date,' she had told the girls, 'but I'm certainly not planning to talk to Matthew about custard creams all night!'

The girls plonked themselves down on the floor around Polly's chic, Balinese-style coffee table to eat their pizza. 'Oh God, I'm almost too tired to eat,' said Jaz, slumped on a cream beanbag, a vision in a beige-and-lime print shirtdress. She was permanently exhausted these days, ironing tights at *Gloss* magazine by day and mixing cocktails in a trendy Soho bar by night to pay the rent; that was on top of her late night at the Blast launch, which had indeed turned out to be a blast. But she, too, had an important date pending. Adam, the complete sweetie, had put in a good word for her with Astrid, fashion guru at Aristo PR for the assistant's job. Jaz had offered her services faster than you can say 'mood-boosting bracelet' and an interview had been set up.

'No pizza for me, thanks,' said Kate, who was sporting a seaweed face-pack and a fetching flowery shower cap (having just applied a deep-conditioning treatment to her new power bob). Tomorrow she wanted to shine – and not just on the career front. 'It's unlike you to turn down carbohydrate, Kate,' said Chrissie, smiling sweetly and flicking back her long, blonde hair. Kate gritted her teeth.
'How much longer is Chrissie going to be living under the same roof?', she wondered. Out loud, she said: 'I wish you wouldn't make such a mess

during your temporary stay here, Chrissie.' It was water off a duck's back. Chrissie, to Kate's great annoyance, had taken to performing a nightly one-woman fashion show as she tried to decide what to wear to work the next day. She was loving her new job at Devastation Records. She had to compete with the Damien Hirst fish tank in reception for attention, but she was certain she'd be 'discovered', even if it did mean getting up an hour earlier than she would have liked to do her hair and make-up in the mornings.

Chrissie had decided to make a special effort for tomorrow's date with Steve. True, it was Laura who Steve was interested in – Chrissie's (blind) date was supposedly Steve's old school friend. But she was planning to win Steve's undivided attention by the end of the first course. After all, Laura, wearing her TV researcher's uniform of combats and trainers, was no match.

But Chrissie almost dropped her slice of pizza when Laura picked up a pink slingback from under the table and asked to borrow it. Laura didn't give two hoots about tomorrow's date. As far as she was concerned, Steve was ghastly. Anyway, she only had eyes for John, the elusive assistant producer. She'd agreed to go on this date partly because she was a clever networker who rarely turned down invitations, but also because she was planning to trial-run a whole new look (Chrissie and Jaz must be getting to her).

'So Pol, what are you up to tomorrow?' asked Kate. 'Oh, nothing much. Harry's out with the boys so I'll probably watch TV,' was the reply. Secretly, Polly was very excited. Simon had phoned that afternoon to say that he would be in London for the weekend and had invited her to dinner. Needless to say, she had already booked a manicure and leg wax, and a blow-dry with Charles for Saturday morning.

praise the updo

Whether it's a simple top knot or a polished French pleat, an updo can make you feel really pulled together and glamorous. Putting your hair up can give you a big confidence boost. Not only is it an instant fix for a bad-hair day, but if you are going out after work, an updo can help you to switch instantly into out-to-play mode. And don't think that putting your hair up is only for formal events. Björk-style twists and scrunched-up top knots are great for clubs and hot, sweaty atmospheres. (It's one way to ensure that your hair stays up as long as you do!) If it's a really big date, nothing beats going to the salon to have your hair put up professionally. But even at home, mastering the art of the updo is a cinch.

the high pony

Ponytails, worn high on the head, Versace-style, can look great for evening. The effect can be super-sexy, rather than sweet and innocent. An added advantage is that a high, tight ponytail is renowned for its instant face-lifting effects. This style works best on unwashed hair because it is easier to work with.

you need

Smoothing brush • covered elastic band or piece of wet string • matt hair grip • serum or glossing spray

1 For a sleek look, brush your hair, pull it back and fix it on top of your crown with a covered elastic band. Alternatively, use a wet piece of string, which will contract as it dries, holding the hair in place securely.

2 Cover the band with a scarf or take a piece of hair from the ponytail, wrap it around the band and secure it underneath with a matt hair grip.

3 Smooth the hair with serum or glossing spray.

the chignon

Chignons – as worn by Audrey Hepburn, Eva Perón an Grace Kelly – are just *so* chic. They're also a great w to look groomed on a bad hair day.

you need

Gel or hairspray • a covered elastic band or a piece of string • matt hair grips • a hairnet if your hair is layered • serum

1 Apply a little gel or hairspray to smooth back the hair and sweep it into a ponytail at the nape.

2 Twist the hair around the elastic band or string as if making a figure-of-eight shape to create a neat bun.

3 Fasten with grips and cover with a hairnet to keep the ends neat. Or leave off the hairnet and pull a few strands forward to soften the look.

4 Smooth a couple of drops of serum over the surface for extra shine.

french pleat

Arguably the the most elegant way to put your ha up – think of Catherine Deneuve's neat French ple in the film *Belle du Jour*.

you need

Medium or firm setting lotion • hairdryer • matt hair grips • hairspray

1 Set or blow-dry your hair loosely, using a mediur or firm setting lotion. (Continues on page 137.)

2 Gently run your fingers through your hair to break it up.

3 Twist the hair up the back of the head and, holding it tightly, secure it in place using matt hair grips.

4 Spray the hair with hairspray to hold the style in place.

5 For a modern take on the classic French pleat, splay out a few ends from the top section to give the style a slightly dishevelled finish (left).

spiky twists

This funky hairstyle works best on medium-length hair. It is a great look for clubbing and parties and is actually a lot easier to do than it appears. Make sure, though, that this style complements the shape of your head and face.

you need

Comb • strong-hold hairspray • matt hair grips

1 Gently backcomb the hair and spritz it all over with a strong-hold hairspray.

2 Take random sections of hair, about 4 sq cm (1½ sq in) in size, and twist them tightly from the base to the ends. Keep twisting each section until it coils back against the scalp forming a top-knot.

3 Using matt hair grips, pin the twists securely against the head, allowing the ends to work themselves loose to create a spiky effect. It's a good idea to cross the grips as this will give maximum support and hold.

4 Continue in this way until the whole head is covered with top-knots.

5 Gently tease and splay out the ends of the hair to create a spiky effect (see right).

top-knot scrunchies

This is a similar style to the spiky twists (below left) but end result is a head full of neat little top-knots.

you need

Comb • strong-hold hairspray • matt hair grips • firm-hold wax

1 Follow steps 1 and 2 for spiky twists.

2 Secure the top-knots firmly to the scalp using matt hair grips as before, but make sure that the ends of the hair are neatly tucked under.

3 To finish, apply a little firm-hold wax to each scrunchie to smooth down any stray hairs.

... polly tries a funky updo

Polly leaves the other girls downstairs and retreats to her boudoir for a bit of peace. She sits down in front of her dressing-table and tries out some of Jaz's new glittery eyeshadow in preparation for her date on Saturday. (Jaz, in true form, had left her make-up strewn all over the bathroom.) She's dying to tell the other girls about sexy cyber-suitor Simon and their little snog in New York, but she knows it isn't a good idea. She feels so guilty about

Harry and anyway, both Jaz and Chrissie are terrible at keeping secrets. Still, she tells herself, there's no harm in having dinner with Simon as he passes through town en route to Geneva. The eyeshadow looks a little out of place with her layered, shoulder-length blonde hair. Polly feels like throwing caution to the wind. After all, on Saturday she'll be off-duty and for once not wearing a neat little suit. Absentmindedly, she twists a section of hair around her finger and pins it to

the crown of her head (as seen in one of Jaz's copies of *Gloss*). The effect is very funky and very un-Polly, but she rather likes it. She carries on twisting random sections of hair, allowing the ends to work themselves loose, creating a spiky effect. By the time she's finished, the effect is more funky urban chick than frumpy City banker. The added advantage is that if she bumps into anyone she knows on her illicit date, they almost certainly won't recognize her.

updo dos
and don'ts

DON'T try and put up newly washed hair as it is just too slippery and floppy to handle.

DO soften a chignon or bun by loosening some wisps of hair around the face, otherwise the overall effect can appear a bit harsh.

DON'T try anything to create a style that is too complicated or too structured so that it looks as though you've tried too hard. (Ivana Trump's beehive is not the look to aim for!)

DON'T use hairpieces for the first time on a big date. It's best to experiment with them beforehand. Your hairdo slipping into your soup is not going to make a good impression.

DO remember to backcomb the roots of your hair. This will set a firm foundation for the perfect updo.

DO use accessories. They are perfect as a quick cover-up for a not-so-perfect updo.

DO use coloured hair mascaras to brighten up selected pieces of hair.

DO carry a handbag-size can of hairspray and some matt hair grips with you at all times to rescue your updo in an emergency.

DO use an invisible hairnet around a bun to keep the hair in place, especially if your hair is layered or has straggly ends.

DON'T try too hard. Sometimes the quickest and messiest updos look the best.

DON'T use accessories that are too heavy as they will pull down an updo and ruin the look.

DO make the most of long hair if you have it. There are times when bigger is definitely better.

HAIR SNIP

FOR SALON-STYLE HAIR AT HOME IN AN INSTANT: TO MAKE LONG HAIR LOOK FABULOUS IN NO TIME AT ALL, HERE IS A QUICK, SIMPLE HAIR-UP TRICK. SECURE THE HAIR IN A PONYTAIL HIGH ON THE CROWN USING A COVERED ELASTIC BAND. AS YOU PULL THE PONYTAIL THROUGH, CATCH THE ENDS IN THE BAND TO FORM A LOOP. ARRANGE THE ENDS INTO A FAN SHAPE AND SEPARATE THEM WITH GEL. IT DOESN'T MATTER IF THE STRANDS WORK THEMSELVES LOOSE, THIS ONLY ENHANCES THE LOOK.

corn-rows

This is a very groovy look, but be warned: you need to have an elegantly shaped head as this can be quite a severe hairstyle. If you want to try this style for the first time, it's a good idea to go to a salon and have it done professionally, but if you are good at plaiting, try doing it using the following instructions.

you need

Comb • sectioning clips • snag-free mini elastics (coloured bands or hair beads, optional) • matt hair grips

1 Section the hair into lots of small 'rows' from the forehead to the nape, holding them out of the way with sectioning clips.

2 Starting at the forehead, plait each section into a mini French plait, keeping them tight against the scalp.

3 Secure each plait with a mini elastic band. Different coloured bands or beads can be used for a quirky effect.

4 If you find it too difficult to plait, just twist each section tightly instead and secure it using matt hair grips.

bun rings

A speedy, easy way to put long hair up is to use a bun ring (you'll find them in most large pharmacies).

you need

Smoothing brush • snag-free elastic band • hairspray • hairdryer (optional) • bun ring • matt hair grips • tail comb • light glossing spray

1 Using a smoothing brush, scrape your hair back into a low ponytail, securing it at the nape with a snag-free band. Spray hairspray onto a huge make-up brush and smooth it over the surface of the hair to control any stray ends.

2 Place a bun ring around the ponytail and secure it with matt hair grips.

3 Start to wrap the hair around the bun ring section by section, and secure it with matt hair grips.

4 Carry on until you have completely covered the bun ring and all the sections are neatly secured in place.

5 When the hair is secure, gently pull a few wispy strands out of the bun using the end of the tail comb and finish by spraying with a light glossing spray (right).

6 Stick a feather or decorative hairpin through the bun if you want to add drama (left).

fake an updo

Even if your hair is only medium-length or shorter, it is still possible to create an impressive up-sweep by weaving a little practical magic with a hairpiece.

mane piece

The foolproof way to secure a hairpiece is to take a 2-cm (¾-in) section of your own hair at the crown or below. Twist it into a knot and pin it. Then place the comb of the hairpiece into the knot and pin it on either side. For a really slick finish, try the following.

you need

Snag-free elastic • matt hair grips • weft of hair approximately 1 m (3 ft 3 in) long • fine hairpin

1 Sweep your hair back into a tight ponytail at the nape and secure it with a snag-free elastic.

2 Attach the weft of hair, wrapping it once around the base of your ponytail and securing it with matt hair grips.

3 Take a small section of the weft and wrap it around the ponytail a few times to disguise the join and secure it underneath with a fine hairpin.

uptown girl

This is a look that is guaranteed to turn a few heads.

you need

Hot rollers • hairspray • bun ring • matt hair grips • hairbrush • long diamanté necklace (optional) • hairpins

1 Set your hair on large hot rollers and lightly spritz it with hairspray.

2 When the rollers are cool, take them out and let the curls droop slightly.

3 Pile the hair through a bun ring and use matt hair grips to hold it in place.

4 Backbrush the hair loosely, causing it to 'candy floss'.

5 Sweep the hair randomly around the head, letting tendrils fall across the face. Make sure you retain some height on the crown and hide the bun ring (right).

6 If you want to accessorize, push the hair back and drape a diamanté necklace over the front of the hair, securing it with hairpins (left).

dressing updos

Accessories and hair make-up are just as effective for adorning an updo as they are for dressing up loose hair. Everything from glitter slides and beaded hair grips to feathered combs and a diamanté tiara can add drama and glamour to even the most understated chignon, pleat or twist. An updo, however, does open up new accessorizing opportunities: beaded hairpins, decorative chopsticks and feathers are all winners.

stencilling

To add even more oomph to an updo for a big night out, try the following stencilling technique.

you need

Stencil • washable body paint • narrow paintbrush • glitter powder • hairspray

HAIR SNIP

ALWAYS CHOOSE YOUR ACCESSORIES TO MATCH YOUR OUTFIT AND YOUR MOOD. IF IT'S A BIG NIGHT OUT, GO BIG, USING FLOWERS – EITHER REAL OR FAKE – FEATHERS AND COLOURFUL BEADS. IF YOU JUST WANT TO BRIGHTEN UP A DULL OUTFIT, GO SMALLER AND MORE UNDERSTATED.

CHOOSE STURDY ACCESSORIES THAT ARE TOTALLY SEALED AT THE ENDS. THERE IS NOTHING WORSE THAN A GLITZY ACCESSORY BREAKING HALFWAY THROUGH THE NIGHT, OR NOT BEING ABLE TO REMOVE ONE AT THE END OF IT.

1 Choose your stencil design to work with your overall look. You can either buy a pre-cut stencil from a home-decorating store or make your own by drawing or tracing your design onto a piece of stiff paper and cut it out with a craft knife.

2 Position the stencil on the hair and gently dab on the paint with the brush until you have filled in the design. Then dab a little glitter powder onto the wet paint. Make sure you hold the stencil very still to avoid any smudging or a blurred outline.

3 Carefully remove the stencil and blast with hairspray to set the design (see page 149).

it's a wrap

Ribbons and cords look stunning wrapped around updo, but you do need a lot of height.

you need

Hairdryer • blow-drying spray • comb • hairspr • matt hair grips • cord

1 Roughly dry the hair using a blow-drying spray, which is ideal as it is not too heavy.

2 Tip your head upside-down, letting all th hair fall forwards. Lightly backcomb the hai to give it volume and spray it with hairspray

3 Use a matt hair grip to attach the end of the cord to the hair at the nape, then start wrapping it around the backcombed section. You will get a better hold if you do this randomly.

4 Tie the cord around the top section of th hair and secure it with a grip (see page 150

Kate kicks off her power heels with relief and collapses onto the hideously patterned hotel bedspread. God, playing the

... kate does day-into-night hair

art of Miss-Get-Ahead-At-Work is so exhausting. It's 7 pm and the conference has only just finished. Several times during the day's coffee breaks, she had tried to get Matthew to listen to her idea for marketing the new low-fat biscuit brand, but to no avail. All he was interested in was whether she had managed to take down all the minutes. Oh well, there's always this evening to further her career ... Damn, is that really the time?

She's got less than half an hour to get ready. Preparing to jump in the shower, Kate pulls back her hair swiftly into a ponytail, catching the ends in a covered elastic band to form a casual updo. Glancing in the mirror, she realizes that her emergency shower-do actually looks quite good. It's just as well, as she doesn't have enough time to wash her hair and wear it down – it would take hours to preen all those unruly curls into some

sort of shape. Feeling refreshed and revived from the shower, she climbs into her slinky black evening dress (her favourite floral dresses were just too country bumpkin to cut it on the career front, she's decided). Spiking out the ends of her impromptu updo, she pulls a few strands of hair around her face free to soften the final effect and dabs on some glitter gel. Kate is ready to be the belle of the Crunch ball.

... big date night

'Come on, Laura ... it's 8 o'clock and we're late,' yelled Chrissie, pacing up and down the hallway. She looked fabulously lean and willowy in her silvery sequinned jeans and black halterneck top, her hair pulled into a high, Versace-style ponytail. The girls had arranged to meet at home and then take a minicab into town for their double date. But what was Laura up to? She never took longer than ten minutes to get ready, while Chrissie usually took two hours. 'She's probably doing sit-ups or something,' thought Chrissie, knowing Laura's passion for working out.

'I'm coming,' replied Laura, as she negotiated her way down the stairs in Chrissie's elegant pink slingbacks. Chrissie swayed on her stiletto spikes. In place of the usual combats, Laura was wearing a scarlet skirt embroidered with flowers and a stretchy pink top. Her hair looked softer and more flirty than usual and she had little rosebuds clipped into it. 'Wow,' said Chrissie, somewhat taken aback (and, if truth be known, rather piqued) by the unexpected competition. She had never seen Laura looking this good. 'Oh, by the way, Steve phoned earlier to change the venue to Cirque instead of Rush.' Laura shrugged her shoulders as she wondered if Steve's friend could possibly be as dreadful as Steve.

Meanwhile, over at the offices of Bartrum Inc. Bank, Polly was in a panic. Simon had arrived from New York a day early and had called that morning to ask if she could make dinner this evening. She should have said no. Instead, she'd rushed out at lunchtime to buy a new slinky black dress (well, what were bonuses for?). Now she was in the bathroom getting ready. She hadn't had time to wash her hair this morning, thanks to Chrissie hogging the bathroom. So she resorted to her favourite bad-hair-day fix and pulled her blonde hair back into a sleek chignon. Five minutes later she was hailing a cab in the street outside, 'Can you take me to Cirque, please?'

Chrissie stalked into the downstairs bar at Cirque followed closely by Laura who, for someone more used to wearing trainers, had gained command of her kitten heels remarkably quickly. Steve was waiting at the bar alone, wearing leather jeans a fake tan and a smug expression. 'Well, hello girls,' he practically drooled over Laura.
'Where's your friend?' asked Chrissie, sharply. She wasn't going to be able to divert his attention away from Laura if there were only three of them.
'Right behind you.' Laura looked over her shoulder and practically fell over.

Standing behind them was ... John – the object of Laura's desire. Yep, Steve's single friend and Chrissie's blind date was none other than gorgeous sexy, elusive assistant TV producer, John.

Upstairs, Polly walked through the door of Cirque her heart pounding – she wasn't sure whether it was passion or guilt, but she certainly hoped she wouldn't bump into any of Harry's friends. She could already see Simon, waiting patiently at corner table. He looked heart-stoppingly gorgeous Aaggh! What would they talk about? He hadn't mentioned their little tryst in his e-mails – maybe he'd gone off her? Polly still wasn't sure if the tone of this dinner was to be work or pleasure.

Chrissie, meanwhile, was losing patience. Steve wasn't paying her enough attention. Still, Cirque seemed to be packed with good-looking men. 'Time to go walkabout,' she thought. 'Perhaps to the ladies loo upstairs to fix my lipstick.' Swinging her slim hips through the restaurant doors, she suddenly saw a very familiar face. It couldn't be – yes, it was. Polly was sitting opposite a completely lush man who looked devastatingly attentive as he kissed her hand 'Polly,' said Chrissie eyeing up Simon suspiciously 'what are you doing here?'

holiday hair

Holiday's are a great time to experiment with new styling ideas and products, but can be damaging to the hair if you don't look after it properly. A change of climate – whether hot and dry, humid or cold – can cause all manner of hair disasters, from fading colour to split ends. Holiday Hair shows you how to get your hair in peak condition before and after your trip, and provides lots of fantastic styling ideas, whether you're heading for the ski slopes, the beach, a spa retreat or a city.

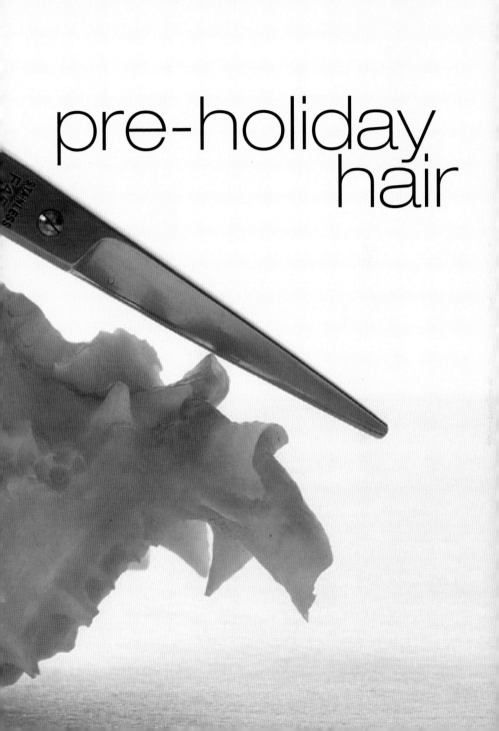

pre-holiday
hair

morning after the big date night

'**So how long** have you been seeing him?' asked Chrissie, the girls' house guest from New York (who now seemed to be a permanent fixture, having originally planned to stay for a month). She'd been dying to know all the details since spotting 'perfect' Polly with a gorgeous man in Cirque the night before. The girls were draped across the sofa in their sitting room, feeling worse for wear after their big night out.

'Since New York,' Polly admitted. She'd been bursting to tell the girls about her cyber-suitor, Simon, since their affair had started. And now the secret was out. 'Are you planning to tell Harry?' demanded Chrissie. How ridiculous of Chrissie to take the moral viewpoint, thought Polly. If she'd met someone as perfect as Simon she wouldn't be letting him go in a hurry. 'I'm going to tell him at dinner,' answered Polly. 'Though I have to say, Chrissie, I thought you'd support me on this. Simon's everything I've been looking for in a boyfriend, everything Harry isn't. I'm sure he's the one.' 'How about finishing one relationship before you start another?' Chrissie snapped.

Chrissie was smarting with jealousy. Despite her careful preening and fabulous outfit, Steve had barely noticed her. It was obvious that his attention was fixed on Laura. To make matters worse, Steve's friend John, who was supposed to be Chrissie's blind date, turned out to be Laura's work colleague. It was clear from John's enthusiasm and Laura's flirting that they were keen on each other. Chrissie could hardly believe it – two gorgeous men competing over Laura! Chrissie was used to being the centre of attention and yet last night no one had seemed interested in talking to her. Now she could tell that Polly was bursting to talk about Simon and how they had got together, but Chrissie's hurt ego had got the better of her. The details of Polly's affair would have to wait; the two girls fell into a tense silence.

Upstairs, Laura was just waking up. She lay in be[d] for a while thinking over every detail of last nigh[t]. She'd nearly fallen off her kitten heels when she discovered that Steve's single friend was John, th[e] sexy assistant TV producer at work. The rest of th[e] evening had been fantastic. Her flirty hairstyle a[nd] feminine clothes had done the trick – not only ha[d] Steve been drooling over her all evening, but Joh[n] had made it clear that he was interested in mo[re] than work chat. In fact, he'd asked for her numb[er] before she left the club and she'd watched hi[m] write it on a card and carefully tuck it into h[is] wallet. Laura was delighted with herself. She[']d played her part perfectly all night: flirty an[d] interesting but just that little bit unavailable at th[e] same time. She smiled to herself. 'He'll call me[,]' she thought, 'he won't be able to resist.'

In her executive hotel room, Kate was suffering wi[th] a hangover and crushed confidence. She'd felt so su[re] of herself when she was getting dressed for th[e] Crunch Ball the night before. Entering the ballroom[,] she'd caught the eye of her boss, Matthew, and h[is] double take had given her a rush. 'You look really [...] great,' he'd managed to say. But just as she'd begu[n] her carefully planned, bright and engaging conversatio[n,] Rachel, a leggy brunette from the sales division, ha[d] slipped her arm through Matthew's and pulled hi[m] towards her. Cutting into Kate's conversation mi[d] sentence, Rachel had looked her up and dow[n] patronizingly and said, 'You don't mind do you Kate[,] Matthew and I have got some important figures t[o] discuss.' Without a backward glance, Matthew ha[d] walked off with Rachel giggling on his arm. The re[st] of the evening had been a complete nightmare. Kat[e] had decided to drown her sorrows with complimenta[ry] champagne, and she'd looked hot and dishevelled b[y] the time she reached her room later that night.

going away

ach year we look forward to our holidays and dream
 sun-drenched days, relaxation and the chance to
dulge ourselves, pushing our holiday budgets to the
nit. We buy new clothes, cosmetics and perfume to
ok our best while we are away and often leave our
aircare to the last minute. Foreign travel – whether it's
 a hot destination for some sun, sandy beaches and
ear blue sea or to the mountains to enjoy fresh air
d crisp snow – will always be good for recharging your
atteries, but rarely good for your hair. On holiday you
e going to be miles away from your usual hair salon
ad the creature comforts of your own bathroom.
owever laid-back you might want to be on holiday, it's
ely that there will be moments when you want your
air to look its best. And whatever the climate of your
estination, you will probably be outside your usual
vironment and, as a result, your hair will be under
tack from weather that it's not used to.

ur hair, unlike your skin, has no natural defence
stem. The ultraviolet (UV) rays of the sun, even on a
latively cloudy day, beat down on your head and dry out
ur hair. UV rays create free radicals, which attack the
air within the hair shaft as well as on its surface. The
gments within the hair (which give hair its colour) are
amaged by the sun, and daily exposure breaks down the
air's strength, causing a loss in colour intensity, shine
d vitality. So, when you are away, you should try to
ink of your haircare routine in the same way as you do
ur skincare routine. When you go on holiday, you pack
 cleanser, moisturizer and sun-protection and after-
n lotions for your face; your hair needs similar
eatment. Shampoo, conditioner, sunscreen for hair
d a styling product should all make it into your wash-
g. You should condition colour-treated hair after every
ash – at home or on holiday. Uncoloured hair should be
nditioned when you are away to prevent damage from
e new environment. Remember, you cannot over-
ndition your hair. Just choose a conditioner to suit your
air type, be it fine and flyaway or thick and curly.

cold climate

Cold weather makes hair very brittle and can cause
dryness. The effect on the hair is just as if you were to
climb into a refrigerator and cool your hair down
extremely quickly – it leaves it weakened and vulnerable
to damage. Low temperatures can also cause static or
flyaway hair and this is a particular problem for fine hair
types, especially those with poker-straight hair. Many
people tend to rough-dry their hair, leaving it slightly
damp, and simply tie it back before going outside –
a definite no-no for hair in the cold. Keep your hair
well conditioned if you are spending time in low
temperatures and, whenever possible, wear a hat to
keep your hair from exposure to the cold.

fine hair
Use a gentle, everyday shampoo and a light, leave-in
conditioner to keep the ends of your hair protected.
In extremely low temperatures, always use a heat-
protection spray before styling, and work some serum
sparingly through the ends of the hair after blow-drying
to seal the hair shaft and lock the moisture in. If you
find your hair becomes static, spray a little hairspray
onto your brush and smooth down the flyaway hair.

curly hair
A good conditioning treatment after shampooing
your hair helps to keep your tresses shiny and well
conditioned. Again, a heat-protection spray is a must,
plus serum after blow-drying to keep the hair hydrated.

frizzy hair
This tends to be much drier than other hair types. Use
a leave-in conditioner after shampooing and take a
deep-moisturizing mask with you on holiday to give the
hair an intensive treatment at least twice a week. A heat-
protection spray and hair serum will keep the moisture
locked into your tresses and keep the elements out.

humid climate

Whatever your hair type, your hair swells and expands when it's wet and behaves in the same way in a humid climate, where the air is full of moisture. Humidity will make hair fluffy and, if it's prone to curling, it will cause frizziness. All hair types will benefit from a pre-holiday conditioning treatment in the salon to nourish the hair shafts and seal the cuticles. Preventing excess moisture from entering the hair shaft in a humid climate is key.

fine hair

This tends to get weighed down by the moisture in the air and looks flat and limp. Just as with other hair types, you need to block out the humidity if you can. A pre-holiday salon treatment will help to reduce split ends and close the cuticles that allow water to enter the hair shaft. Use a light leave-in conditioner on your hair while you are away (apply it from mid-way down the length of your hair to the ends) and seal the ends of the hair after blow-drying with a serum. Be careful not to use too much serum on fine hair – a blob the size of your thumbnail is more than enough. Hairsprays are a great SOS option for a bad-hair day in humidity – they instantly hold down the cuticle of the hair and prevent moisture from entering the hair shaft.

curly and frizzy hair

Sealing the outside of your hair – the cuticle – is the only way you will minimize the candyfloss look while you are away. A pre-holiday deep-conditioning treatment is a must. Make sure you pack a creamy leave-in conditioner for your trip and use it religiously every morning. Using an anti-frizz serum will help bring unruly curls to heel. It coats the hair shaft with silicone, not only sealing the cuticle but also weighing the hair down a little. If your hair is really frizzy, try working some serum through it while it is still wet before blow-drying. This should add some weight to the curls and seal the cuticles so that your hair does not absorb water, swell and frizz again as it dries. If you decide to go with the flow and make the most of your curls while you're away, mix gel and serum together in the palm of your hand and apply it throughout the hair to give the curls extra definition and shape.

hot, dry heat

The sun can strip the hair of its natural oils and a heat will only intensify the problem. Just two weeks the sun without protecting your hair can weaken h cuticles, with peeling, breaking and split ends becom a problem. The sun's UV rays attack the melanin pigme that gives hair its colour, as well as the keratin, t protein fibres, within the hair shaft that provide streng and elasticity. A weakened cuticle leaves hair vulnera to dehydration and the colour bleaches and fades. S exposure also encourages free radical activity in the h shaft. The cells of the hair are damaged, as the fr radicals cause premature ageing. Deep-conditioni treatments are vital before travelling to a hot clima especially for chemically treated hair. However, the o way to protect your hair 100 per cent from sun dama is to keep it out of the sun – a hat is the best option.

fine hair

Pack a gentle daily shampoo and a light leave conditioner with UV protection. A sun-protection spray th contains a UV filter will help screen the hair from the s and sea water if you are sunbathing on a beach. Reap the spray through the hair after each dip in the sea.

curly hair

Pack a gentle moisturizing shampoo to cleanse your h daily, plus a creamy leave-in conditioner to help gua against excess dryness. If you are sunbathing, apply a su protection spray or oil that contains a UV filter to redu sun damage to the hair, and reapply it regularly, just you would suntan lotion to your face and body. Take nourishing hair mask with you to deep-condition your h

frizzy hair

Your hair tends to be dry anyway and needs extra care dry heat. As before, use a sun-protection spray or oil your hair during the day and make sure you apply a ri leave-in conditioner with UV protection to your hair ea morning before going out in the sun. Apply a hair ma to your hair at least every other day during your holic – you can leave it on overnight for an intensive treatme if your hair becomes very dry in the heat.

holiday hair enemies

All weather and climate changes bring environmental aggressors that are damaging to your hair. The perfect holiday setting – sun, sea and sand – provides the key elements that damage your hair. For hair to be sleek and easy to style it must be well moisturized – a difficult task when you are exposed to extreme heat (and conversely extreme cold). A trip abroad is the perfect time to spend some money on good-quality hair products to protect, condition and bring out the best in your hairstyle.

rain

A sudden shower will always catch you unaware, so, unless you have an umbrella or hood to cover your hair and prevent it from getting soaked, dive into the nearest café and sit out the storm in comfort. The haircare rules for rain are similar to those for a humid climate: block out the excess moisture or pay the price. If you become drenched in a sudden downfall, only to watch the sun come out afterwards, be careful about letting your hair dry too quickly. The sun's rays will heat up the hair shaft, drying out the hair and causing it to lighten. You wouldn't try to blow-dry your hair when it is dripping wet – you would towel-dry it first and then rough-dry it before styling it properly – and the same care should be taken after a rainstorm. Carry a travel-sized bottle of conditioner in your beachbag or rucksack and if you get caught in a storm, smooth a little conditioner through your wet hair to help protect it while it dries naturally. Comb it through to leave it looking styled or tie it back loosely to look instantly groomed. If you have frizzy hair, smooth some anti-frizz serum through it, pull it back into a ponytail and let it dry naturally. When it's nearly dry, brush it straight, secure with hair grips and leave it until it is bone dry. You should be left with soft waves rather than corkscrew curls.

sea

Salt is your enemy here as it roughens up the surface of the hair, leaving it dull, damaged and porous. If your hair is colour-treated, the combination of sea salt and sun damage will make your colour fade rapidly. A leave-in conditioner (which contains UV protection) goes some way to protect the hair, as it coats the hair shaft and acts as a physical barrier to the salt. If you are happy to slick your hair back while you lie on the beach, use a sun-protection oil or wax on the hair to hold the cuticle down and prevent the hair shaft from being damaged. Always wash the salt out of your hair thoroughly at the end of each day.

chlorine

Chlorine is extremely bad for the hair, especially when combined with the sun's rays. When your hair is wet it acts like a sponge and is highly absorbent. So when you are in a swimming pool and wet your hair, chlorine enters the hair shaft, leaving it looking dull, dry and brittle. The best way to protect your hair is to wet it in the shower before heading for the pool and cover it liberally with a leave-in conditioner to coat the hair shaft, preferably one containing a UV filter to give extra protection from the sun's rays. Alternatively, try applying a non-water-soluble hair wax, which will act as an effective barrier (this is more suitable for shorter hair). Wash your hair thoroughly every day after swimming.

Tie your hair back while you are on the beach as sand will roughen the surface of the hair. Give it a good, long rinse at the end of each day to get rid of any sand, then condition your hair, squeeze out excess moisture with a towel and gently comb it through.

air travel

Ever gone on a long-haul flight and left the aeroplane with your hair glued to your scalp or crackling with static electricity? The air pressure in the cabin, coupled with the dry air, high altitude, nylon seat covers and magnetic field in the aeroplane causes even thick hair to become static. It's possibly the worst atmosphere for hair. Tie your hair back and place a silk headscarf over your headrest to minimize the static effect on your hair. Always travel with your hair free of styling products so that it can breathe. Take a small can of hairspray or a mineral-water atomizer in your hand luggage, plus a small comb or brush. Spritzing water over your head rehydrates and revitalizes your hair during a long-haul flight. Control static hair at the end of the flight by spraying a little hairspray onto your brush and brushing it through the hair to minimize flyaway strands (this will work just as well in cold weather when hair can also become static). Drink plenty of mineral water during the flight – it's important for your skin as well as your hair.

A cold, strong wind will cause some dryness. Keep your hair well conditioned and tie it back to keep it groomed and in place.

sun

Sun dehydrates the hair. The overlapping cuticles, which protect the centre of the hair shaft (its cortex), peel and break as they dry out in the heat. The cortex is made of keratin, a fibrous protein, which gives the hair its strength and elasticity. The sun's UV rays damage the hair by breaking down its protein structure. When the outer hair cuticle becomes damaged, or porous in the case of chemically treated hair, it's all the more easy for the sun's rays to enter the cortex causing dehydration and fading the hair colour. Sun exposure also increases free radical damage, causing premature ageing in your hair, just as in your skin. Look for products with built-in UV protection – everything from your conditioner to sun-protection spray for the hair. Or simply use regular sun-protection lotion on your scalp to prevent burning.

nner with **Harry** goes badly. espite his recent lack of nthusiasm for their relationship, e's furious that Polly is calling off. His male ego is taking a attering and he isn't going down lently. With his voice getting eadily louder, he argues through e main course and storms out efore coffee arrives. Polly pays e bill quietly and goes home.

Vaiting for her on her laptop is message from Simon: 'Come way with me. Flights and hotel ooked – leaving Saturday. Surprise estination. Pack for the sun.' omance is exactly what Polly's een dreaming of, but sense tells er that this could be moving too ast. How can she take time off ork? City deadlines are non-egotiable. More importantly, her ghlights are in desperate need f attention – her natural colour's nowing through and Polly, ever ractical, has no intention of flying

.. polly's last-minute hair prep

ff for a romantic week with a bad ase of root regrowth. Her answer, he decides, will be governed by hether she can get a last-minute ppointment with her colourist, arolyn, before they're due to fly.

Jext morning, Polly arrived at vork early, determined to keep er mind off Harry (she does eel guilty for hurting him), and ff Simon's exciting plans. The alon receptionist gives her an

appointment for a half-head of highlights and a hair mask. (It pays to be a regular customer.) Her decision has been made for her and, since she's taken so little of her annual leave, her boss is in no position to refuse her holiday request. Polly e-mails her reply to Simon: 'Great idea. See you at Heathrow. Can't wait.'

At the salon, Carolyn puts a few foils along Polly's parting and

around her hairline to even out the root regrowth. 'The sun will lighten your hair, Polly,' she says, 'so I'm not going to put too many highlights in now. Let's book you in for a cut and colour for your return and we can take a look at your hair colour then,' she advises. She also applies an extra-rich, creamy conditioning treatment to Polly's hair to give it a remoisturizing boost. Polly is now ready for her trip.

hair prep

In the run-up to your holiday, make time to book a consultation with your hairstylist and colourist to discuss your particular hair needs. Your salon can provide professional conditioning treatments that will keep your locks in top condition throughout your holiday and minimize the damage caused by various environmental aggressors while you are away. Ask your hairstylist to recommend an at-home intensive conditioning product and make a conditioning treatment part of your weekly haircare routine in the month before your holiday. This will give your hair a head start when it is faced with a change in climate.

Choose your haircare products carefully. Look for shampoos, conditioners and styling products that offer UV protection if you are going to be outdoors and in the sun on your trip. Make the most of the latest travel-sized versions of your favourite products – not only will they save valuable space in your luggage, they will also be convenient to carry around with you for on-the-go styling during the day. A great alternative is to decant your favourite products into small plastic travel bottles (available from good pharmacies) so you can travel light.

cut

A good haircut will compensate for a more casual holiday styling routine, so that you still look well groomed. Your hairstyle should be able to hold its shape even if you opt for minimal styling while you are away and dispense with the daily blow-drying, leaving your hair to dry naturally. Get your hair in shape by having a simple cut that requires only minimal effort to look good. A gently layered style, for example, will laterally fall naturally into place and needs very little maintenance. Warn your hairstylist that you are going on holiday so that he or she can work your cut into an easy-to-manage shape and leave enough length to trim away any split ends on your return.

cutting considerations

Type of holiday If you are travelling in a hot climate or will be particularly active on holiday, you may want the option of wearing your hair up. Plan ahead – if your hair is short to medium length decide whether to let it grow longer so that it can be tied back.

Consult your hairstylist He or she might recommend having a few layers cut into your hair (to add shape) so that it looks good and is easy to style on holiday.

Be realistic You may want to inject some freshness into your look, so, as well as buying a few new holiday outfits, get advice from your stylist on different ways to style your haircut. Holidays are a great time for experimentation and trying out different products.

colour

Book a consultation with your colourist before your holiday. You may want to have your roots retouched or your colour revitalized with a tint so that it looks perfect for your trip. To look fabulous while you are away, have your hair colour done two to three weeks before you go, so that it is fresh and your hair has time to settle before your trip. However, depending on your destination and the climate there, your colourist may advise waiting for a full-colour treatment until your return. Blonde highlights will go even lighter in the sun, so warn your colourist if you are heading to the heat. It may be better to put a few tints around your parting and hairline, rather than using bleach on your hair before your trip. Similarly, lowlights and tints will fade in the sun, so your colourist might suggest a revitalizing colour treatment on your return, rather than before you go. Remember, chemically treated hair is porous and more vulnerable to the elements. If your hair is colour-treated or permed it will lose moisture faster than untreated hair and will need extra care while you are away.

blonde hair

Ask for a quarter-head of highlights rather than the full head of highlights before a trip to a sunny climate. This will colour the area around your face, on top of the crown and at the sides to refresh your colour. The sun will lighten your colour further while you are away. If you have lots of very light highlights through your hair, have a few natural blonde lights put through before your holiday as they will go lighter in the sun, so you will not damage the condition of the hair so much.

red hair

Have your colour done two to three weeks before your holiday and ask your colourist to mix a corresponding vegetable tint to take with you to refresh the red during your stay. Alternatively, use a coloured mousse (in the same shade as your hair) to refresh any light or brassy highlights. Test the colour on a white tissue before putting it on your hair, as some colours can be a bit misleading.

brown and dark hair

Ask your colourist to lighten a few tips of the hair around your face before a holiday to the sun. It looks naturally sunkissed and will lighten a little while you are away, leaving flattering highlights close to your skin.

colour considerations

1 Use a shampoo and conditioner formulated for colour-treated hair. You need moisturizing products that gently cleanse and condition the hair shaft. Deep-cleansing shampoos will lift colour tint out of the hair faster, so stick to gentle, daily formulas. Many shampoos and conditioners for colour-treated hair now contain UV protectants that can reduce sun damage.

2 You will always need a hair-colour treatment after your holiday, so if in doubt, wait until your return.

3 The ultimate protection for your hair colour is a hat or headscarf. Don't forget to tuck the ends of your hair into the hat as they are vulnerable to the sun if left exposed. The only way to avoid colour fading is to keep your hair out of the sun altogether.

hats for different face shapes

To properly protect your hair you need to keep it covered from the elements or out of the sun altogether. S wearing a hat is the most realistic option for shieldin your hair while you are out and about. A baseball cap c headscarf will be better than nothing, as both cover you scalp and, to some extent, your hair. The best solutior though, is a hat with a decent brim that will shade you face and neck along with your hair. If you are sitting i the sun, always tuck the ends of your hair up into you hat – they are the driest part of your hair and the mos vulnerable to damage from the environment.

oval faces

Virtually any hat shape will suit an oval face, as the proportions of the face are even. Choose one that you feel confident wearing, otherwise it will sit unused in your hotel room during your trip.

round faces

Balance a round face with a ha that has a good, high crown an a decent brim. A short crown an small brim will make your fac look more round.

long faces

A hat that has a wide brim will offset the length of a long face. Choose one with a low crown – a high crown will make the face look even longer.

heart-shaped faces

Most hats will suit a heart-shape face, although a medium-size brim (rather than a wide brim) w help to prevent the jaw line fro looking too narrow.

ack at the house after her
terview at Aristo PR, Jaz is
acking her overnight bag. Fashion
R guru, Astrid, has offered Jaz
job provided that she makes a
ood impression on a key client
Paris. They are catching the
urostar train that evening and
aving dinner with one of Paris's
op young designers. Tomorrow
hey have a meeting with a buyer
Galleries Marais department
tore to help the designer introduce

Jaz sprays some shine enhancer
through her hair and brushes
her thick, dark locks into a neat
high ponytail. Then she smooths
down loose hairs with a natural-
hold hairspray. She looks chic
and ready for business. Jaz
packs Kate's hair straightener.
She knows she looks much more
stylish with long, sleek hair and
it usually has a natural kink when
she wakes in the morning. Kate
had reminded her that she'll find

complimentary shampoo in
her hotel bathroom, so she
just packs her own quick-rinse
conditioner, as she hates using
heavy conditioners on her hair.
She finds a travel-sized bottle
of mousse, which she pops
into her washbag. It will help
her to style her hair quickly
in the morning. She also packs
her multipurpose smoothing
brush, which she can use
when she blow-dries her hair.

.. Jaz's trip to the fashion capital

s collection. Having spent months
acking up clothes in the fashion
epartment at *Gloss* magazine,
az is finally entering the fashion
rcuit for real. She has to perform
ell – and look directional and
tylish for the next 24 hours.

lothes are not a problem – she
as Chrissie's wardrobe to choose
om as well as her own. She
ecides to travel in black, low-
ung trousers and take Chrissie's
amel leather skirt and pointed,
igh-heeled boots, which look
reat with skirts and trousers.
couple of tops and her new
nee-length military coat will cover
ll the options. What to pack for
er hairstyling needs proves more
f a problem. She's fairly certain
he hotel will provide a hairdryer,
ut should she take hers in case?
az calls Kate to ask her advice.
Why don't you borrow my hair
traightener? Don't forget to
ack a travel plug – a three-pin
ne won't work in Paris,' she says.

holiday hair tips

maintain the condition

Look after your hair on the plane – you don't want to damage it before you even get to your destination. Use a serum to protect it and spritz it with mineral water to rehydrate. Remember, salt water will dry and dehydrate the hair, so use a detox shampoo to cleanse away the salt and then condition with a moisture mask. If your hair does start to dry out, brush it every night with a natural-bristle brush. This will encourage natural oils, which will moisturize dry hair. While you are on holiday, remember to eat healthily and drink lots of water. Both your body and your hair will benefit.

protect, protect, protect

Ideally, wear a hat or headscarf to protect your hair from the sun's rays, but remember that heat can also damage the hair, so condition it well to prevent it from drying out. When you are not wearing a hat, make sure that you protect your scalp. It is part of your skin, so use sun-protection lotion to prevent it from burning.

special treatment for coloured hair

If you have coloured hair, seek advice from your stylist before you travel. You may need to have your colour done before or after your holiday, but either way it is very important that you get the right advice to achieve best results and maintain good condition. Delicate blonde hair will suffer if you spend lots of time in smoky clubs while you are away – serum will coat the hair shaft and act as a barrier, while detox shampoo will cleanse away any stains. If you have naturally brown hair that shows signs of fading in the sun, rinse beer through it to add depth and gloss, and then rinse well with water.

accessorize

Take a collection of coloured ribbons with you for dressing up your hair for going out. Ribbons make great accessories, are easy to pack and are available in lots of colours and materials that can be matched to any outfit. Hair fragrance is also very useful for freshening up the hair when you don't have time to wash it.

travel kit

brush and comb

A wide-toothed comb can be used on wet hair and is essential to banish holiday tangles. You should also pack a small all-purpose brush to cope with all your styling requirements.

hair accessories, grips and bands

Pack at least one stunning hair accessory for your holiday. If you're going to the sun, a tropical-flower clip would be ideal, whereas a diamanté comb or sparkly slides might be appropriate for a city jaunt. Matt hair grips are useful for pinning your hair up (in a twist or chignon), and covered elastic bands are the perfect quick-fix solution to most haircare problems – just tie your hair back. If you like to leave your hair loose, a wide fabric or zigzag headband is great for keeping it off your face.

products

If you're going on a beach holiday, take a gentle, everyday shampoo to wash the sun, sea and sand right out of your hair, while a detox shampoo is extra-cleansing for hair that is exposed to city grime or smoky clubs. A good conditioner with a UV filter is the key product for holiday hair. Don't expect to return with your hair in decent shape without it. In addition, pack an intensive hair mask for the ultimate moisture boost. Also essential if you are going to sunny climes is a sun-protection spray. As with suntan lotion, you should reapply this regularly throughout the day, especially after swimming.

travel plug

This is essential if you are heading abroad, since no hairdryer, straightener or electric curling tong will fit a foreign socket without it.

holiday babes

getting away from it all

Things were going from bad to worse in the marketing department at Crunch Biscuits. Matthew was too preoccupied with the latest Crunch Creams campaign to listen to Kate's idea for marketing the new low-fat biscuit. Kate found herself buried by a seemingly endless stream of marketing figures that she had to input into the system. Feeling demoralized, she opened her second pack of chocolate-chip cookies of the day and tucked in. Gazing around the office she saw all of her colleagues concentrating hard on their work. 'They're all so driven,' she thought to herself. 'And I'm stuck in this dead-end job with a boss who barely acknowledges me.' Picking up her bag, she quietly left the office and headed towards the nearest travel agent.

Five minutes later she was clutching an airline ticket. 'I'm suffocating in my life, and I'm going nowhere,' Kate thought. 'Polly's got her high-flying job in the City, Jaz's new job means she'll be surrounded by glamorous designers and fabulous-looking models, and Laura's working on a fascinating new real-life documentary.' The daily grind at Crunch Biscuits seemed mundane in comparison. 'I'm going to take charge of my life,' Kate resolved. 'A two-week yoga retreat in India is just what I need. I am going to relax and find my inner strength.' She walked slowly back to the office, sat down at her desk and filled out her holiday request form. Matthew barely read it as he signed it, and mumbled something about organizing adequate secretarial cover while she was away. Kate let his indifference wash over her – at last she had something to look forward to.

That evening at the house Jaz and Chrissie were in a restless mood. Polly's sitting room was covered with discarded fashion magazines, open CDs and the remnants of their supper. Laura was in her bedroom with the door closed yet again. She h[ad] been mooning around ever since the night [at] Cirque, was hardly talking to the girls and wo[uld] rush to answer the telephone every time it ra[ng]. Jaz's trip to Paris had given her a taste for t[he] high-life – she was in a full-on party mood. Chris[sie] was still smarting over her lack of success w[ith] Steve at Cirque. She was also a little concern[ed] that her receptionist's job at Devastation Recor[ds] was doing more to enhance her telephone sk[ills] than her career. She was still no closer to be[ing] 'discovered'. 'We need to get away, we need to g[et] some sun,' Chrissie whined to Jaz.
'And how are we going to do that?' Jaz replied. '[We] haven't got any money to spend on a night out, [let] alone a holiday.'

Chrissie knew it was true. Her uncontrollable shopp[ing] habit took care of any spare cash; she never cou[ld] resist a new pair of shoes or the latest handba[g]. Jaz's unpaid work placement at *Gloss* magazine h[ad] cleared her savings account and her new job [at] Aristo PR put a considerable strain on her ba[nk] balance. She had been shopping every lunchtim[e] since she'd started work, trying to put together [a] fashionable wardrobe for the office. 'Well, we [both] have our Visa cards,' said Chrissie, who had whipp[ed] hers out of her wallet and was waving it in the air[.] Jaz looked nervous. 'Do you think we should?' she sa[id]. 'You're only young once,' laughed Chrissie. 'Let's [go] and party in Ibiza. We can book it tomorrow.'
'You can book it on the Internet now,' said Laura, w[ho] had just walked into the room. 'I've just booked mi[ne].'
'Your holiday?' shrieked Chrissie and Jaz togeth[er].
'Would you like to tell us where you're goin[g]?' demanded Jaz.
'And who with?' added Chrissie.
'The jungle in Sumatra, and John, as a matter [of] fact,' Laura replied coolly.

beach babe

There's not anything much you would rather be doing than lying on the beach and soaking up the rays. If you're not curled up on a sun lounger engrossed in the latest blockbusting romantic novel, you're strolling along the beach, taking a dip in the sea or enjoying some waterskiing or windsurfing when you have a burst of energy. You're a high-maintenance girl on the hair front: all that sun, sea and sand are going to make your hair drier than the Sahara Desert. That ice-filled cocktail from the beach bar won't help matters either.

hair solutions

Work water-resistant suntan lotion or a sun-protection hair product into the roots of your hair and spread it evenly across your scalp and around your hairline. Your head can easily be burnt through your hair by the sun and your hairline is a particularly sensitive area. If your scalp does get burnt, the hairline tends to peel first – which is not a great holiday look.

The best way to style your hair is to keep it simple during the day. Tie it back into a slick ponytail if your hair is long enough, or just comb it back once you've applied your sun protection through the roots if your hairstyle is shorter. Remember, though, wearing a hat is the best protection for your hair.

Make sure that you wash your hair thoroughly at the end of each day to rinse out all of the salt, sand and sun-protection product, then give your hair a good condition. If you have the time, apply your conditioner or hair mask and spend 20 minutes relaxing before rinsing to give the hair a real boost. Let your hair dry naturally if you're having a relaxed evening, or twist it up into a chignon if your hair is long enough for instant chic. Blasting your hair with a hairdryer or styling it with straighteners and curling tongs while you are in a hot climate is going to make dry ends worse – so try to limit your use of them to evenings when you want to look really special.

holiday tool kit

- Daily-wash shampoo
- Heavy-duty conditioner
- Nourishing hair mask
- Hair-protection spray with UV filter, or suntan lotion to use on your scalp
- Snag-free elastic hair bands
- Wide-toothed comb
- Headscarf or hat
- Styling product to suit your hair type

braid it

This is a fun, sexy look for beach parties and barbecues, but it is time-consuming to achieve and you need to set aside plenty of time to do it properly.

you need

Approximately 30 lengths of 5 mm (¼ in) ribbon • sectioning comb • scissors for trimming ribbon

1 Starting at the front of the hairline, use a sectioning comb to neatly section off a piece of hair about 2.5 cm (1 in) square.

2 Tie a length of ribbon securely around the section of hair at the roots.

3 Twist the section of hair all along its length, from the roots to the ends.

4 Tightly holding the ends of the twisted section of hair with one hand, wrap the ribbon neatly around the hair, crisscrossing as you go. Tie the ribbon securely around the ends of the hair and trim any excess to tidy.

5 Continue sectioning, twisting and braiding all over the head in the same way.

ɔeach bunches

his is an easy style which you can do in no time at all
efore hitting the local nightspots. It's fun, cute and
endy – and perfect for clubbing, too.

ou need

ectioning comb • two snag-free bands • matt
air grips • glossing spray or light-hold hairspray

Use the comb to part the front section of the hair to
ne side. Then take the parting diagonally back to the
pposite corner in the nape of the neck.

2 Comb the hair neatly into two ponytails and
secure them with snag-free bands, making
sure they are tight at the roots. Position the
ponytails wherever you like, but for a quirky finish
place them at different angles to each other.

3 Taking each ponytail in turn, twist the hair loosely and
vind it around the base of the ponytail. Secure the ends
f the hair into the ponytail base using matt hair grips.

4 Finish by lightly spraying the hair with a
glossing spray or light-hold hairspray to hold
down any stray ends.

mohican pony

lolidays are all about relaxing and having fun, so if
ou're feeling daring, let out the punk rocker in you and
-y this unusual style, which is guaranteed to turn heads
vherever you go. You can either use coloured bands
nd cord or, as here, stick to neutral tones.

ou need

ectioning comb • snag-free bands • light wax •
∋ngths of cord

Starting at the front of the head, take a section of hair
om ear to ear, comb it up smoothly and tie it securely
vith a snag-free band.

2 Take the next section of hair, from above
the ear on each side, comb it neatly to the top
of the head and gather in the remainder of the
last ponytail. Start to secure with the band as
before, but this time leave the hair in a loop.

3 Repeat this process, working your way down the
head to the nape of the neck. Leave the last section as
a ponytail and smooth it with a light wax.

4 To finish, wind lengths of natural cord
around the bands to disguise them.

HAIR SNIP

WHILE YOU ARE ON HOLIDAY, DON'T
BE SCARED TO TRY OUT SOMETHING
DIFFERENT WITH YOUR HAIR –
REMEMBER, YOU PROBABLY WON'T
EVER SEE THESE PEOPLE AGAIN.
YOU CAN GET LOTS OF GREAT
IDEAS FROM MAGAZINES

flower girl

Before you start, make sure the hair is free of any kno
– you do not have to have clean hair for this style, but
will be more comfortable if you comb out any tangles

you need

Sectioning comb • clip • matt hair grips • flowe

1 Section off the top part of the hair and clip it temporarily
out of the way, leaving the back hanging loose. Gently pu
the sides and back section into a loose ponytail and twist
it up to the crown, holding it in place with matt hair grips.

2 Unclip the top section and loosely twist
it back randomly, securing it with matt grips.

3 Finally, add a fresh or fake flower and grip it in plac

french plait

You will probably need the help of a friend to do th
and get the shape perfect, but once you have got it,
will probably last for a couple of days, and can b
accessorized for the evening.

you need

Tail comb • snag-free band • hair grip • light-hol
hairspray

1 Start by sectioning a 2.5 cm (1 in) square piece of hai
parallel with one eye. Using a tail comb, start creating a
spiral shape, running behind the ear towards the nape.
While you are sectioning the hair, get your friend to star
plaiting tightly against the scalp.

2 Carry on working towards the crown area
keeping an even spiral while doing so.

3 When all the hair is plaited, secure the ends using a
band and secure the tail of the plait to the top section with
a grip. Finally, use a little hairspray and the pointed end of th
tail comb to push any flyaway hair into the plait to neaten.

snow white

u can hardly wait to get to the mountains. During the
y you keep your hair off your face with a warm hat or
adband that covers your ears as you zoom down those
untain slopes. By night, you can be found enjoying
e après-ski in a dark, smoky bar.

air solutions

e snow reflects the sun's rays, making them even more
werful, so protect your hair by using a good, leave-in
nditioner with a UV filter. Keep your hairstyle simple,
orty and chic – glamour girls look out of place on the
opes. The cold makes your hair brittle and static, so keep
and or slide in your pocket to pin back flyaway hair.

oliday tool kit

Daily-wash shampoo
Leave-in conditioner (with UV filter)
Snag-free elastic hair bands or hair slides
Hair serum and hairspray (to help combat static)

ski chic

ker-straight hair is the ultimate in sophisticated cool.

ou need

ow-drying spray • paddle brush • hairdryer •
raightening irons • light water-based wax

Spritz the hair with blow-drying spray and use the
ush to blow-dry it straight, section by section. Glide
e hot straightening irons down the length of the hair.

2 Finish with a light wax for extra gloss.

ce queen

is style is a modern take on movie-star glamour. It's
irky yet sophisticated, and easier to achieve than it looks.

you need

Comb • large heated rollers • snag-free band •
2 hairnets (to match your hair) • hairpins • hairspray

1 Section your hair on large heated rollers to create
volume and a good foundation to hold the style.

2 Section off the top rectangle of hair, from
the crown to the temples, and sweep the
remaining hair into a ponytail above the nape.

3 Backcomb the ponytail and cover it with a fine
hairnet to form a bun. Secure with hairpins and hairspray.

4 Lightly backcomb the top section and
twist it round, loosely. Secure the shape
with pins and hairspray.

euro chick

Weekend city breaks are your thing. You like the stylish, cosmopolitan look with hair that will take you from chic boutique and café to museums and elegant restaurants.

hair solutions

The pollution and weather are your hair threats, so wash it daily with cleansing shampoo and condition it to put the moisture back in. Carry leave-in conditioner or serum with you in case you are caught in a rainstorm, and use sunglasses to hold hair off your face for a quick fix.

holiday tool kit

- Gentle cleansing shampoo
- Leave-in conditioner (with UV filter)
- Small can of hairspray
- Matt hair grips (to control stray hairs or pin hair up)
- Natural-bristle brush (to help keep hair free of dirt)
- Sunglasses (the stylish hair solution)

daytime sleek

This is the perfect style for city chic and can be ea adapted for a high-glamour evening look (see below

you need

Comb • large heated rollers • flexi-hold hairspr • natural-bristle brush

1 Section the hair and wind it onto large heated rollers The top section should go across to one side, the side should go forwards and the back should go downwar

2 Spritz with flexi-hold hairspray to give maximum hold and leave to cool.

3 Gently take the rollers out and smooth the ha using a bristle brush. If the hair is static, spray the bru with hairspray. Finish by spritzing with flexi-hold hairspr

evening chic

Simply sweep back the sides and backcomb the top.

you need

Comb • large heated rollers • flexi-hold hairspr • natural-bristle brush • sectioning clip • firm-ho gel • matt hair grips

1 Prepare as for daytime sleek, above.

2 Clip the top section of hair out of the wa and, using a firm-hold gel, comb the sides aw from the face and secure with matt hair grips

3 Backcomb the top section at the roots to give maximum lift and grip in place, letting the hair fall loose over the face. Spritz with hairspray to finish.

yoga fiend

ether you're stretching your limbs in a yoga class or lying
ck for a massage, your hair is the last thing you should be
rried about. Go for a natural look – creating big, glamorous
ir is not a part of your holiday agenda.

air solutions

ep hair low maintenance by tying it back casually or
ting it hang free. Pamper your hair as well as your body
apply a deep-conditioning mask, lie back and relax.

oliday tool kit

Shampoo and conditioner
Deep-conditioning hair mask
Wide-toothed comb
Snag-free elastic hair bands and hair slides

mask it

is is brilliant if you need to give your hair a treatment
at will boost its moisture levels and combat dehydration.

ou need

omb • deep-conditioning treatment • snag-free
and • fine hairpins • grips

Comb a moisturizing treatment through the hair, working
ht the way through the length, from the roots to the ends.

2 Twist the top section of hair loosely onto the
top of the head, then pin it in place.

3 Secure the rest of the hair in a ponytail at the nape
the neck , and place a grip above and below the band.

hair treat

en if your hair is in good condition, this treatment is ideal
keeping it out of the way while you pamper yourself.

you need

Comb • deep-conditioning treatment • snag-free
bands • fine hairpins

1 Comb a moisturizing treatment through the hair as above.

2 Make a ponytail in the centre of the head
and plait it, securing the ends with a band.

3 Wrap the plait around the head and secure it in
place with fine hairpins.

HAIR SNIP
TAKE ADVANTAGE OF THE HEAT, WHETHER
IT'S THE SUN OR A STEAM ROOM. HEAT
ALLOWS THE TREATMENT TO PENETRATE
DEEPER INTO THE HAIR SHAFT.

st tropez babe

When you are surrounded by celebrities, rock stars and royalty on holiday, you need a hairstyle that grabs some of the attention for you. Don't be afraid to make an impact with your hair. High-octane glamour is the only way to go – your hair has to be big, bold and full of body to make sure you really stand out from the crowd.

hair solutions

By day you need to look sleek and chic for lounging on the beach and hanging out in cafés drinking cappuccinos and watching the world go by. Stick to simple styles for low-maintenance elegance and remember, less is more for the daytime. Smooth ponytails, neat bobs and understated twists will give you effortless style. But by night, you need to rev up the pace with all-out glitz and glamour – go for big hair every time. The best way to achieve this look is by backcombing or backbrushing your hair, but remember only to backcomb the roots, otherwise you will be left with an uncontrollable bird's nest, instead of St Tropez glam! Remember, too, that all the sun and nightly hairstyling will take its toll on your hair. Whenever you get the chance on holiday, bathe your locks in a nutritious hair mask to keep the gloss and shine in your hair.

holiday tool kit

- Medium-hold setting spray and hairspray
- Medium-hold hair mousse
- Deep-conditioning hair mask
- Covered elastic hair bands
- Brush or comb for backbrushing

glamour curls

This hairstyle is truly 'big hair' like never before. The curls give great volume and texture, and the finger-styling creates a tousled, backcombed feel. This style works best if you have long hair, as the weight of your locks pulls the curls downwards.

you need

Medium-hold setting spray • hairdryer • heate(
rollers • medium-hold hairspray

1 Spritz medium-hold setting spray evenly throu(
damp hair – the weather will determine how lo(
this style will last, so be generous with the spray a(
make sure you cover the hair evenly. Then blow-c(
your hair thoroughly.

2 Make sure your rollers are as hot as they can get. Then, starting at the top of your head, take medium-sized sections and wind them onto your hot rollers.

3 Spray the hair with medium-hold hairspray t(
help keep the humidity out. Leave the rollers to co(
for as long as possible – use this time to put you(
make-up on and get dressed.

4 When the rollers are completely cool, gently take them out and apply some mor(
medium-hold hairspray. Then, using you(
fingers like a comb, pull through the hair t(
break up the curls. (To make the style bigge(
use your fingers to backcomb the hair.)

HAIR SN(
ADD EXTRA BODY TO YOUR STY(
BY MASSAGING STRONG-HO(
HAIR MOUSSE TO THE ROOTS (
THE HAIR WHILE IT IS WET. FIR(
ROUGHLY BLOW-DRY THE HAIR(
REMOVE EXCESS WATER, TH(
WORK THROUGH THE HAIR(
SECTIONS, LIFTING THE ROOTS(
AND AWAY FROM THE SCALP WITH(
VOLUMIZING BRUSH TO GIVE EXT(
BODY TO THE HAIR AS IT DRI(

va-va-voom

...less curly – but equally glam – version of big, big hair.
...is is pure rock-chick-meets-European-princess.

...ou need

...airdryer with diffuser • blow-drying primer •
...ow-drying spray • large velcro rollers • hair-
...pray • natural-bristle brush • light shine spray

...Start by blow-drying the hair using a blow-drying
...imer to give body and 'guts'.

2 When the hair is 90 per cent dry, spritz
it evenly with blow-drying spray.

...3 Using large velcro rollers, wind medium-sized
...ections of hair straight down onto the base of each
...ection. Make sure that you wind the hair in the desired
...rection, otherwise it will be difficult to style.

4 Dry the hair using either a portable
hood dryer or a diffuser. Make sure the hair
is 100 per cent dry, then let it cool right down.

...5 Starting at the bottom and working up, take out
...e rollers, making sure that you do not tangle the hair.

6 Spray the hair with hairspray, then gently
backbrush the root area to create lift.

...Finish by smoothing a bristle brush over the surface
...the hair and spray using a light shine spray.

accessorize it

...e severity of this sleek style is counteracted by the
...etty hair grips, which add instant sexiness and softness.

...ou need

...airdryer • light-hold mousse • paddle brush •
...traightening irons • blow-drying spray • pretty
...air grips • wax

HAIR SNIP
TAKE A HAIRPIECE AWAY WITH
YOU TO ADD INSTANT LENGTH
AND VOLUME TO YOUR LOCKS.
THIS CAN BE ATTACHED AT THE
BACK OF THE HEAD TO GIVE
THE ILLUSION OF LENGTH, AND
THE JOIN CAN EASILY BE DISGUISED
WITH YOUR CHOSEN ACCESSORIES.

1 Start by blow-drying the hair smooth using a light-
hold mousse and a paddle brush.

2 Starting at the nape, straighten the hair
section by section using the straightening
irons. Spritz each section with blow-drying
spray first to protect the hair.

3 Tuck the front sections behind the ear and hold
them in place with your chosen accessories.

4 Finish the ends with wax to add texture.

The pressure of keeping their relationship quiet at work, along with the normal demands of a fast-paced job in TV, has made Laura and John decide to take a break. They are both passionate about wildlife and quickly agree on a ten-day trek in the jungles of Sumatra to see orang-utan in their natural habitat. It's far from a comfort holiday but they both know they'll come back having had an adventure. Laura looks at the clothes and toiletries laid out on her bed and sighs as she lifts up her compact rucksack. Despite her tomboy attitude she can't seem to organize her belongings into vital, possible and unnecessary items. It's early days in her relationship with John and while she won't need kitten heels or a hairdryer, she wants to look attractive and effortlessly cool. She'll be carrying her rucksack from one camp to the next, so she needs to make sure it's as light as possible. A washbag full of products is a definite no: it seems to weigh a ton. She gets tough and singles out four T-shirts, two pairs of shorts, a swimsuit, trekking boots and

... laura's hair-raising dilemma

sandals. She faces the question of cosmetics. A light, frequent-wash shampoo and leave-in conditioner with UV protection are a must. She'll be lucky to find a bucket of water to wash with along the trail and she needs to protect her hair from the damaging rays of the sun. Her cropped hair will dry quickly in the heat, but the humidity will play havoc with her hair and she doesn't want to face John with a bad case of cotton-wool hair. A small bottle of anti-frizz serum should do the trick – she can use it sparingly to give texture to her hair, weigh it down a little, hold her style and stop the ends from frizzing. Suntan lotion, after-sun cream with insect repellent, mascara, toothpaste, a tooth-brush and an all-over face and body cleanser all make it into her washbag. A wide-toothed comb will help keep tangled hair at bay. She's managed to halve her packing in one go.

backpack girl

eedom is a rucksack on your back and a guidebook in
ur hand. Your holiday is far from luxurious, but whether
u're trekking in a jungle or camping on a beach, you'll
 having the time of your life. You have to carry your bag
 your back, so everything you pack must be useful.

air solution

ke away your favourite products in travel sizes to
t down on space and weight. You need a gentle, daily
ampoo to rinse your hair quickly – your bathroom
cilities will probably be basic. Use a leave-in conditioner
 protect your hair from the sun. Take only the styling
oducts you'll need to create a low-maintenance, casual
ok. Hair serums will help prevent frizz if you're in a
imid climate and the easiest quick fix will be to tie your
ir back. Slides and accessories will give instant glamour.

oliday tool kit

Gentle daily-wash shampoo
Leave-in conditioner (with UV filter)
Hair serum and hair wax (to perk up a short hairstyle)
SOS glamour kit: hair grips, accessories and
snag-free elastic hair bands

short 'n' sweet

u do need a textured haircut to create this funky style,
it it's easy to maintain when you don't have much time.

ou need

airdryer • light gel spray • firm-hold wax • hair grips

 Dry your hair using a light gel spray to give lift at the roots.

2 When your hair is dry, mould it into shape,
then work in a firm-hold wax to create texture.

3 Comb the fringe (bangs) back from the face and
ecure it with hair grips.

dreadlocks

Dreadlocks look cool but they can be difficult to comb
out, so be certain you like the look before you commit.

you need

Fine-toothed comb • light-hold hairspray • wax

1 Take a 2.5 cm (1 in) section of hair and gently twist it
from roots to ends, then spritz it with light-hold hairspray.

2 Using a fine-toothed comb, gently
backcomb along the length of the hair.

3 Run wax over the surface of the dreadlock to
prevent it from unravelling.

fresh-air queen

Whether you're walking, mountain biking or horse riding through the hills, your ideal holiday is always in the countryside. Glamour is not top of your list, but practicality is key for your activities. In the evenings you go for a natural look, making the most of your hair with an easy-to-style cut that holds its shape with minimum effort.

hair solutions

Depending on your destination, you're likely to be exposed to sun, wind or rain all day, so protect your hair with a leave-in conditioner. Keeping your hair out of the way will be essential. Use styling wax or an extra-hold gel on short hair to work it back from the face and tie longer hair back. A little hairspray will hold down those loose strands. Gently style your hair in the evenings with the help of a mousse – it'll make your post-shampoo styling quicker and help hold your hairstyle for longer.

holiday tool kit

- Daily-wash shampoo
- Leave-in conditioner (with UV filter)
- Wax, styling gel or mousse and hairspray
- Snag-free bands or grips (to keep hair under contr
- Wide-toothed comb (to keep tangles at bay)

country curls

Just wear plaits by day and unravel them for evening cu

you need

Comb • styling spray • snag-free bands • clip

1 First shampoo and towel-dry your hair; then comb c any tangles and spritz with styling spray.

2 Section the hair into 5 cm (2 in) square sections and plait them tightly from roots to en Fasten with bands and dry the hair in the sun o with a hairdryer, then unravel the plaits. Clip up the top section of the hair and add a flower.

twist and shout

These easy-to-do twists create a relaxed, fresh look.

you need

Hairdryer • blow-drying primer • hairpins • wa

1 Dry the hair using a blow-drying primer spray for extra and hold. Twist the top section of hair onto your crown a secure it with pins, letting strands fall out for added textu

2 Twist the back section up and pin it as before, again leaving strands to fan out.

3 Finish by using wax on the ends to add definition.

Chrissie and Jaz stumble onto the beach, hiding the signs of their hangovers behind dark sunglasses. Having clubbed through the night until 6 am, they haven't had much sleep and they hardly have the energy to do more than put on their bikinis and walk the short distance from their beds to the beach. They spot two free sun loungers and, with a sudden burst of energy, run down the beach to grab them.

Jaz and Chrissie are having a fantastic time. The night before they'd made an extra effort to show off their newly acquired golden tans by wearing matching micro miniskirts and sparkly lycra tops which they'd bought specially for their holiday. (They knew they'd attract more attention if they wore identical outfits.) Jaz had decided to straighten her hair to a glossy sheen by spritzing on some anti-frizz serum and carefully running the straightening irons

along each section from the roots to the ends. She'd then pulled back the top and secured it with a sparkly diamanté clip. Chrissie had scraped her hair back into a high ponytail and secured a platinum-blonde hairpiece to its base, covering the join with a strand of her own hair. The length of hair down her back almost reached her waist and she looked fantastic. 'Aren't you ready yet?' she'd called to Jaz, 'We've got some partying to do!'

Chrissie and Jaz party on ...

'That's me done for the day,' laughs Chrissie, as she spreads her towel across the lounger, flops down and closes her eyes. Jaz quietly begins her daily ritual of sun protection. She smooths suntan lotion all over her body and then squeezes a blob of leave-in hair conditioner onto the palm of her hand and mixes some suntan lotion into it. She works the mixture over her scalp and around her hairline. 'You are ridiculous Jaz,' teases Chrissie. 'I can't believe you bother doing that every morning.' 'Just protecting myself from the sun,' replies Jaz, as she combs her hair back into a loose ponytail. 'You ought to wear a hat, with your blonde hair and fair skin,' she warns, uncharacteristically sensible. 'This holiday is about being wild and crazy, Jaz,' says Chrissie. 'I don't remember you playing safe last night ...'

club bunnie

From Ibiza to Aya Napa, you can be found dancing the night away from dusk until dawn and then sleeping off your hangover in the sun by day. This type of holiday is really going to put your hair to the test. You'll be exposing it to the sun's rays during the day and smoky environments by night. And not only that – you'll also be subjecting it to heavy-duty styling to create glamorous looks with a high wow-factor.

hair solutions

As well as giving your hair a daily cleanse and detox, you also need to condition it on a daily basis to keep it from drying out during your high hair-maintenance holiday. Your focus is going to be on creating sassy, funky styles for the evening, so make sure you pack your favourite strong-hold styling products to give extra staying power to your hairstyle. A rich, conditioning hair mask will help to keep your hair moisturized, so that you don't return home with dried-out, stressed tresses – use it at least twice a week on your trip.

holiday tool kit

- Detox shampoo
- Leave-in conditioner (with UV filter)
- Hair mask
- Extra-hold styling products: mousse, hairspray, wax and serum (depending on your hairstyle)
- Selection of pins and grips for stylish updos
- Snag-free bands (for beach hair during the day)
- Glitzy hair accessories for instant glamour, such as flowers, butterflies, feathers and gemstones

funky hair

Funky hair is what every club bunnie needs. The idea is to look hip, sexy and effortlessly cool. This dishevelled look is easiest to create on short and medium-length layered styles. You just need plenty of firm-hold mousse to make sure your style lasts as long as you do.

you need

Firm-hold mousse • hairdryer (with diffuser) • several plastic hair combs • glossing spray

1 Generously apply firm-hold mousse, making sure all the hair is completely covered.

2 Gently blow-dry the hair until it is 80 per cent dry using a diffuser or the slow setting on your hairdryer.

3 When the hair is 80 per cent dry, place combs firm into the hair as needed, positioning them so that the ha fans out in different directions.

4 Once you are happy with the shape your hair is creating, continue drying your hair until it is completely dry; this will ensure your hair stays up all night.

5 Finish with a good spritz of glossing spray, which will make your hair extra shiny.

tips for club bunnie

Use lots of products to give your ha substance and hold – there is nothir worse than a collapsed hairdo halfwa through the nigh

Use snag-free bands and matt ha grips – these will hold the hair in plac without damaging

If you have very long or thick hair, try keep it tied back. This will keep you co and prevent your hair from getting swea and collapsing when you're dancin

high pony

his is a sleek, high-glamour look that will look great
nd help keep you cool when you are dancing.

ou need

airdryer • light-hold mousse • paddle brush •
traightening irons • comb • 3 snag-free bands
hairpins • glitter and gel (optional)

Blow-dry the hair smooth using light-hold mousse
nd a paddle brush. Then straighten the hair section
section using the straightening irons.

2 Divide the hair into three horizontal
sections, securing each with a snag-free
band. Then wrap a strand of hair around
the base of each bunch to disguise the
band and secure it with hairpins.

3 Backcomb the base of each ponytail to make it
and away from the head and, for extra drama, use
el to stick chunky glitter along one side of the head.

chopstick twists

is excellent hairstyle is great for a big night out, and
rprisingly quick to achieve (see overleaf).

ou need

air grips • firm-hold hairspray • chopsticks

Taking a 2.5 cm (1 in) square section of hair, twist it
htly from ends to roots, letting the hair wind down on itself.

2 Wind the ends of the hair tightly around the
base and secure it with a hair grip.

3 Continue by winding sections of hair all over. When
u have twisted all the sections, apply firm-hold hairspray.

4 Accessorize the twists with chopsticks (as
shown here), or with flowers, feathers or beads.

ponytail tips

Make sure ponytails are firmly secured to
prevent them from slipping or loosening.
Hold them in place with snag-free bands
or wet string, which contracts as it dries,
holding the hair even more tightly.

To give a neat, slick finish, wrap a small
section of hair around the ponytail base
to cover and disguise the hair band.
Secure the section of hair in place
using a matt hair grip.

Use chunky glitter to accessorize your
hairstyle. This can be fixed in place by
applying a little strong-hold gel to
the desired area before adding the
glitter. Finish with a strong-hold
non-aerosol hairspray.

holiday hair
quick fixes

Take a bottle of fresh tap water with you to the beach to rinse the sea salt out of your hair throughout the day. Remember to do this, and then to reapply leave-in conditioner (with a UV filter) or sun-protection spray to your hair (and suntan lotion to your face and body) after every dip in the sea.

2 Keep a travel-sized bottle of leave-in conditioner or a travel-sized can of hairspray in your backpack or beach bag at all times in case of emergencies. You can use either one of these products to seal the ends of your hair or slick down stray ends for a quick style fix.

3 Keep a thick, cotton-covered hair band handy to tie back your hair for on-the-spot grooming. As an extra precaution, smooth a little conditioner over the band to help prevent you from snagging or tearing your hair when you remove it later on.

4 This is a great quick fix for naturally curly hair. After washing your hair as normal, apply a firm-hold styling mousse evenly through your hair. Taking one small section of hair at a time, twist each one from the roots to the ends. Carry on until your whole head is covered in twists of hair. Then dry it slowly using a diffuser on your hairdryer, being careful not to disturb the twists of hair while you dry them. When your hair is dry, unwind the twists and you'll be left with a head full of spiral locks.

5 Apply hair-protection lotion as often as you would apply your regular sunscreen to your face and body. The golden rule is to reapply. One spritz in the morning does not give day-long protection.

6 If it all gets too much, simply push your hair back from your face and hold it in place with your sunglasses. Wearing your sunglasses as if they were a hair band is a stylish – and fail-safe – quick fix.

7 If you have short hair, take styling wax with you on holiday. You can use it to rework your hairstyle into funky chunks in an instant if you get caught in the rain or are suffering the consequences of a humid climate.

8 Tie back long hair at the nape of your neck, rather than scrunching it up on the top of your head while you are out and about. This way you will avoid exposing the ends of your hair to the sun (important even on a cloudy day when the UV rays will still be strong), thereby preventing them from becoming dry and brittle.

9 Sun-protection body lotions and oils can be used on your hair (in small amounts only) to protect your scalp from the sun. Apply a few drops through your hair and work it onto your scalp by massaging with your fingertips. Don't forget to apply sun protection to your ears, as they will be exposed to the sun, especially if you tie your hair back.

10 Give yourself a cool sporty look and slick back those loose ends with a wet-look sun-protection gel containing a UV filter (go for the no-hold type). This will give your hair extra protection if you are swimming and sunbathing a lot; it works well on long hair if it is being tied back, as well as on short hair, and can be reapplied regularly during the day to keep the sun-protection factor up.

get back
into shape

exotic experiences

On her third morning, Kate woke in her tiny room at the ashram in Kerala. It was only 6 am and yet she felt completely awake and healthier than she had in ages. Her daily routine of yoga classes, meditation and cleansing Ayurvedic treatments were doing the trick. She felt more confident about herself. Her vegetarian diet and daily exercise regime had given her that sought-after smooth stomach. She knew she looked good, despite the fact that she hadn't bothered to put on even a stroke of mascara since she'd arrived. The only thing that didn't agree with the Indian climate was her hair: it had frizzed into bouncy ringlets and there was little Kate could do about it. She surprised herself by not caring in the least.

Stretching happily, Kate jumped out of bed and threw on some linen drawstring trousers and a white, fitted T-shirt. She grabbed a towel, slipped on her flip-flops and set off for her morning yoga lesson. 'Good morning,' said a voice behind her. It was Luke, a tall, suntanned guy who was living at the ashram for six months' training to become a yoga teacher. 'Did you sleep well?' he asked Kate. 'Fantastically,' she replied. 'I haven't felt this rested in ages. I won't know myself after two weeks here.' 'I thought I'd join your class this morning,' said Luke. 'Great,' said Kate, trying to contain her delight. She hadn't met anyone like Luke before; he was calm, intelligent and genuine to everyone he met. She was fascinated to find out more about him, what had drawn him to the ashram and why he wanted to become a yoga teacher. Perhaps breakfast after their yoga class would give them the chance to chat.

Polly was sitting on the hotel balcony at a table covered with a crisp linen tablecloth, enjoying a breakfast of fresh pineapple and papaya while gazing out over a sparkling, turquoise bay. Simon had just taken a shower and walked out onto t balcony wrapped up in a white towelling robe. looked wonderful, and Polly had never felt happi London, her City job and Harry all seemed a world aw 'I've organized a day out on a speed boat for we're leaving at 10.30 so there's no need to rus he said as he stroked her hair. 'Then tonight we having dinner at a rather special seafood restaura one of the other guests recommended to me. in the next bay along from the hotel, looking over a deserted beach.'

Back in their minimalist hotel room after a s drenched day on the boat, Polly washed the salt a suntan lotion out of her hair and thought about wh she was going to wear for dinner. She wanted to lc chic but relaxed, so she pulled a turquoise dress of the wardrobe and slipped on some kitten-h mules. Her golden skin looked fantastic agair the turquoise of her dress. She spritzed a lit volumizing spray through her hair, relieved th she had remembered to buy some mini-sized h products in the airport before the flight. Polly th blow-dried her hair with a curling brush to put so volume into her blonde locks, before twisting her h up into a casual but so chic chignon. She pinned h hair into place and looked at herself in the mirror. dash of bronzing powder across her cheeks, a lit sparkly eye-shadow, mascara and soft pink lip glc were all she needed to enhance her healthy glc She was ready for her evening with Simon.

After a short drive along the coastline, Polly a Simon were seated at a secluded table looking c over the golden sand. Simon ordered a bottle Champagne, raised his glass to toast their eveni and then reached across the table for Polly's har 'Polly,' he said, looking serious, 'I've got somethi I want to talk to you about ...'

SOS hair repair

f you are concerned in any way about your hair once you get back from your holiday, go to your hair salon for a consultation. This is normally free of charge and gives you the chance to talk through the condition, cut and colour of your hair with your stylist and colourist so that they can advise the best plan of action for post-holiday haircare.

cut

The quickest way to get holiday hair back into condition is to cut out all the dry, split ends that leave it looking dull. Once hair has been cut back into shape, it will look sleek and shiny without much extra effort. Remember to book an appointment before you go away, so that you can dash into the salon on your return. If your hair is dry and damaged, your stylist may have to cut away up to 1 cm (½ in) to get it back into condition. But if you've spent time conditioning your hair while you were away and it's in good shape on your return, your stylist can just snip away the split ends without taking any length off your hair.

colour

Once you are back from holiday, continue to treat your hair with conditioning treatments. This will even out porosity, maintain the condition and ensure that your next colour treatment takes evenly. Give your hair a weekly detox shampoo to remove the build-up of chlorine and salt water on the hair shaft. Have a good look at your colour once you get home. You may love the sun-kissed highlights around your face and on the tips of your hair, so take a photograph of it. That way, your colourist has a reference and can re-create the look if you want holiday glamour put back into your hair at a later date. If your hair has gone too light, your colourist can add some deeper lowlights or apply a colour gloss to tone down the overall colour, make it look more natural or take it back to the colour it was before your trip.

holiday tips for coloured hair

A great way to start a hair-repair regime is with a scalp and head massage, as it stimulates the secretion of natural, moisturizing oils.

Use a cleansing detox shampoo, which leaves the hair ultra-clean and revitalized, then apply a deep-conditioning treatment to replace moisture and even out the porosity of the hair.

Colour glossing treatments rejuvenate hair colour, and add shine and condition, without drying it out.

There are products that help prevent colour fade, so splash out on these before you go away – it'll be cheaper than a repair job when you return.

Back from their holiday, Jaz and Chrissie are feeling far from refreshed and rejuvenated. They have partied through the night and sunned themselves on the beach all day long for the entire week, and are now well and truly in need of a post-holiday overhaul. They're sitting in the kitchen assessing the damage. Chrissie has overdone the sunbathing and she's suffering the consequences – she's burnt her scalp, her hair looks dry and brittle, and she's beginning to peel around her hairline. Jaz is worried about split ends. Despite her careful attempts to protect her hair, all the heat from the sun, together with her nightly hairstyling regime has left the ends dry. 'Let's finish off our holiday with a pampering session,' says Jaz. 'We've spent so much already, a little extra on a trip to the salon won't hurt,' agrees Chrissie. 'Great tans, girls,' says Charles as he greets them at the salon. 'But your hair is in distress!' 'Do whatever you can,' sighs Jaz, as the girls sit down in front of the mirrors for their consultations. Charles decides that both girls need to have an intensive deep-conditioning treatment to put the moisture

... jaz's and chrissie's bad-hair day

back into their hair and revitaliz the condition. Then he cuts just the ends off Jaz's hair to get rid of all the split ends without losing the length. Chrissie finds that she needs to have a bit more taken off her hair as the ends have got so dry. 'You need to have some honey-blonde tints put through your hair Chrissie,' says her colourist, Carolyn. 'Your hair's been bleached by the sun and it's too hard on your skin tone,' she advises. 'I'm in your hands,' says Chrissie.

Three hours later, Jaz and Chrissie leave the salon feeling more rested than they have in the whole of the last week. The hair is looking sleek, glossy and full of body. 'We should do this more often,' says Chrissie as the head for a designer clothes shop for a spot of window shopping. 'I think I could just about get used to it,' laughs Jaz.

hair treats

here are a number of really effective treatments you
an use to replenish the moisture levels of dehydrated
air, encourage growth, improve strength and flexibility
nd restore shine and gloss. You can book in for a
eatment at your salon on your return, do it at home, or,
ven better, while you are on holiday to help maintain
ondition and prevent damage from occurring.

calp treatment

s its name suggests, this treatment stimulates and
evitalizes the skin of the scalp for better, stronger hair
owth. It is usually made up of soothing and moisturizing
gredients that help to prevent itching, flaking and
scomfort. It will encourage the growth of new hair by
ourishing the roots and it also conditions the hair
haft. Scalp treatments are good for all hair types,
articularly if the scalp is burnt or dry after a holiday.

onditioning mask

esigned to be left on the hair for between 3 and 20
inutes, a conditioning mask will hydrate the hair shaft
ith moisturizing ingredients and nourish the hair and
calp without causing heaviness. Conditioning masks
e designed to work most effectively on the damaged
 dehydrated areas of the hair, leaving it nourished and
otected. This is a good treatment to use during your
oliday and on your return, whatever your hair type.

eep-conditioning treatment

ore intensive than a conditioning mask, this hair
eatment literally gets to the root of the problem by
ourishing the scalp as well as the hair itself. It homes
 on damaged areas and delivers intensive moisture
actly where it's needed. This extra-rich treatment is
st for extremely dry and parched hair.

air detox

deep-cleansing shampoo that removes the build-up
 dirt, styling products and pollutants from the hair,
thout stripping it or leaving it dry. This is especially
eful if your hair is looking dull after a holiday or for
lour-treated hair that might need a revitalizing boost.

nutrition

Diet plays a huge part in the health of our hair, and a
holiday is a great time to eat well and boost the body's
vitality with good nutrition. The sure-fire way to make
your hair limp and thin is to skip meals or eat badly.
So what do you need to eat?

diet tips

Do not crash diet before you go away, as this puts
strain on the system and deprives your body of
essential nutrients – the first to suffer will be your hair.

A balanced wholefood diet, with essential fats,
plenty of carbohydrates, protein and fresh fruit and
vegetables will keep your hair healthy and shiny.

The best sources of essential fats are oily fish,
such as sardines and salmon, and vegetable
oils, such as olive and linseed (flax); these will
help to keep the skin and hair in good condition.

Eat plenty of carbohydrates such as brown
rice, wholewheat pasta, pulses and lentils.

Fresh fruit, vegetables and salads provide
antioxidant vitamins, which help prevent
premature ageing in the body and the hair.

Since the hair is made up of protein, you need to
keep your protein levels high by means of your
diet. Fish, chicken, meat and eggs all provide
the best proteins, although other sources
such as nuts, cereals, milk and cheese will
also supplement your intake.

hair supplements

A good daily multivitamin will give you the balance
of vitamins and minerals that your body and hair need
to keep them in optimum condition. The condition
of your hair will be boosted by all the B vitamins,
gamma-linolenic acid (GLA), fish oil, linseed (flax) oil,
antioxidant vitamins including beta-carotene, vitamins
C and E, and the minerals selenium and zinc.

Back at home again, Kate decides to spend spend the last few hours of her holiday relaxing. She has a long shower and then applies a conditioning hair mask to her hair, twists a small towel into a turban on her head and wraps herself up in her dressing gown. Kate makes a cup of tea and then, feeling wonderfully relaxed, she settles down on the sofa to watch a video.

Next morning, Kate wakes early and performs her new ritual of yoga stretches before breakfast. Getting ready for work, she takes a good look at herself in the mirror. Her lightly tanned, glowing skin needs little make-up, so she sticks to mascara and a touch of bronzer. Her curly hair is looking glossy and healthy with flattering golden streaks from the sun. She decides to leave it natural and

simply works some styling crème through the ends to give the curl extra definition. Work, and more importantly Matthew, will have to take her as they find her. If two weeks at the yoga retreat have taught her anything, it's to have the confidence to be herself. Her Miss-Get-Ahead-At-Work act has got her nowhere – perhaps her new-found contentment and inner strength will do the trick

... kate returns home from India

An hour later she walks into the office, makes herself a cup of green tea and sits down at her desk to check her e-mails. Matthew walks past her desk and then stops suddenly. 'Kate, I hardly recognized you,' he gasps. His expression changes from surprise to pleasure. 'You're looking fabulous – where did you go again?' he asks. 'You'd know if you'd bothered to ask,' thinks Kate to herself. 'India,' she replies brightly. 'Well, it's obviously agreed with you,' Matthew says, looking her up and down. Keeping his eyes fixed on Kate as he hands her some paperwork, he suggests they go out for lunch so he can fill her in on the latest marketing project. 'Sure,' Kate replies calmly. She turns back to her computer and there in her e-mail inbox is a message from Luke. 'Got the job at The Yoga Centre in Notting Hill. Will be back in two months. Missing you,' it said.

hair
doctor

my blonde hair looks distinctly green after my holiday. Is there anything I can do?

The reason your hair can go green is because of the blue dye that is used to show up the chlorine in swimming pools (chlorine is, in fact, clear). Highlights make your hair more porous than usual and so the blue dye can penetrate the hair shaft and react with the highlighting chemicals in your hair. Try using a detox shampoo designed to thoroughly but gently cleanse the hair. Or, try applying concentrated tomato juice or tomato ketchup to the hair, as the red colouring should neutralize any green in your hair. If the green tinge to your hair will not budge, you need to go to a hair salon where the stylist will 'deep cleanse' your hair with a mild pre-lightening agent to lift out the colour. Your colourist will then freshen up your original colour.

my hair seems dull, lacklustre an flat after my week away. Why is i looking so bad?

It is possible that your hair has been beaten by t combination of sun damage, chlorine or salt and, if y have been using styling products that contain silica, build-up of product on your hair. On your return fro holiday, use a clarifying shampoo to remove de deposits of dirt and the build-up of styling produc Then book yourself into your salon and ask your styl to trim off all the split ends – the result is immedia Your hair will look sharp, clean and sleek. Your styl may also recommend that you have a revitalizing h treatment while you are in the salon, but the combinati of simple cut and condition should do the trick.

my scalp is dry and flaky after my holiday. Do I have dandruff?

Is more than likely that you have burnt your scalp in the
n while you were away and the skin on your scalp is
eling. Dandruff tends to be more common among
ople who have oily hair, not a dry scalp. So if you have
st-holiday flakes, visit your hair salon for an intensive
ep-conditioning treatment that includes a scalp
eatment to feed the hair as well as soothe and
hydrate the skin on your head. Don't rush for the
arest anti-dandruff shampoo unless the problem
rsists well after your return. If, after a few weeks, you
ll see flakes in your hairline, try using an anti-
ndruff shampoo every other day. When lathered up,
member to leave the shampoo on for a few minutes
allow the ingredients to work, moisturizing and
foliating the scalp. Alternate anti-dandruff shampoo
th your usual shampoo until the problem clears.

I wash my hair every day on holiday, will it be more oily when return home?

is one of the big haircare myths that washing your
ir every day will make it oilier. Using a gentle, daily
ampoo will not leave your hair more oily or stimulate
e sebum glands on your scalp to produce more oil.
ore importantly, washing out the cocktail of haircare
oducts, salt and chlorine that usually comes with a
eak away and putting the moisture back into your
ir at the end of each day with a good conditioner will
ave your hair glossy, well conditioned and healthy.

the ends of my hair seem really dry. Can I use a product to repair my split ends?

Any product that is designed to treat split ends offers only a temporary, cosmetic solution. Split-end products and hairsprays simply hold the ends together until either the hair is brushed vigorously or washed. The only way to get rid of post-holiday split ends is to have them cut off. Your hairstylist will be able to snip the ends away without taking a great length off your hair, provided that you have kept your hair in good condition while you were away.

if I use lemon on my hair while I sunbathe is it a 'natural' way to give me highlights?

Lemon juice may help to bleach hair in the sun as the juice is acidic (although how effective it is remains debatable). But be warned: neat lemon juice is extremely damaging to the hair. It will dry it out while you lie in the sun and your scalp may be left sore and sun-sensitive. The sun will fade your hair colour in a hot climate and this bleaching action damages your hair as it weakens the structure of the cells and causes permanent damage. It's best to forget about lemon juice and leave it to your hair colourist to change your colour and add highlights.

polly's big announcement

The girls were all back from their globe-trotting and, at Polly's request, were having a night in together. Her sitting room was filled with excited chatter as they caught up on each other's news. Polly had called from the office to say that she would have to work until 8.30 but that she would bring supper with her. She had to put in some extra time after her break in the Seychelles with Simon in case anyone at her City firm thought she wasn't taking her job seriously.

'I'm going to open a bottle of wine – does anyone want a glass while we wait for Polly?' asked Jaz.
'Yes, and grab some crisps while you're at it,' ordered Chrissie, who was curled up on the floor painting her toenails with iridescent pink varnish.
'So you survived the jungle and John?' she said sarcastically to Laura, who was showing Kate her photographs of river rafting and orang-utan in the jungle's nature reserve.
'It was incredible,' replied Laura, who was very happily reliving the trip. 'John's thinking of moving into nature documentaries. We were both so taken with the wildlife and we want to raise awareness for the conservation work that needs to be done in the jungle,' she said.
'So you'd actually consider living out there for months, with all those huge insects?' asked Chrissie, shuddering visibly.
'Well, I can see how you'd have a problem living without your kitten heels and your hairdryer,' laughed Kate, 'but Laura's pretty resourceful.'

'I'm home,' yelled Polly, as she headed for the kitchen with a bag full of Thai takeaway. 'Come and have some food while it's hot,' she called to the girls. 'I've got green curry, rice and steam vegetables,' she said as they gathered round. Th each grabbed a bowl of food and took it back in the sitting room. 'Champagne?' asked Polly as s joined them with a large, chilled bottle and glass 'This is pushing the boat out a bit isn't it?' said Lau 'Well, it seems to me that we've got things celebrate,' said Polly, handing the girls a gla each. Polly raised her glass in the air. 'Here's Jaz's new job in the fashion world, and to Lau and John's new venture – let's hope it works ou The girls toasted their future as they drank.

'So let's hear about the Seychelles and Simo demanded Chrissie. An uncontrollable smile spre instantly across Polly's face.
'You really like him, don't you Polly?' asked Ka 'He's just perfect. We had the most incredible tir and the thing is, well, he's asked me to marry hir Polly burst out excitedly. There was a momen stunned silence before the girls shrieked in uniso 'Marry him?' gasped Laura. 'Polly, that's so quic 'I know it seems like a whirlwind romance,' agre Polly. 'I've only known him for a few months but both know it's right and we can't see the point hanging around and waiting. I was hoping you wou all be there for me – as my bridesmaids.'
'Of course we will,' answered Laura quickly.
'Now tell us about the ring – have you chos a huge stone?' asked Chrissie, true to form.

The rest of the evening was filled with weddi talk as the girls debated what Polly should we laughed about hideous meringue dresses a discussed how they should have their hair. L at 23 Havana Road had certainly moved on fast

big day hair

Whatever your choice of **wedding**, think of your hair as your greatest **accessory**. Big Day Hair caters for your every hair need, offering **advice** on identifying the look that best suits your **face shape**, dress and accessories, **tips** for getting your hair in peak **condition** in the run up to the big day, **great** hairstyles for every type of wedding – from boho vintage, **classic** and country to **fashionista**, beach and **rock chic** and ideas for easy **transformations** for the **reception** and going away.

choose
your style

the girls digest polly's big news

'I think I need a drink,' said Chrissie, the confirmed bachelorette of the group, in the light of Polly's announcement. (Chrissie had come over from New York to stay with the girls for a month, but now seemed to be a permanent fixture in the house.)

'Luckily, we have some Champagne,' beamed Polly, who couldn't contain her obvious glee. Jaz, Laura and Kate silently exchanged stunned glances, while they tried to take in the alarming fact that aliens may have abducted and replaced their dear friend, sensible 'perfect' Polly. At last, incurably romantic Kate threw her arms around Polly.

'Oh, I just knew it! This is so fabulous, you must be thrilled!' she squealed excitedly.

Laura, Polly's best friend from Manchester, was a little less enthusiastic. 'But, Polly, you've only known Simon for a few months, how can you be sure?' she asked, frowning. Polly had known that Laura would try to be the voice of reason. Even her own budding love affair with her long-term object of desire, John, didn't seem to have softened her stoic tomboy nature.

'Look, I know you're only concerned for me,' Polly said, flopping down onto the sofa next to Laura and taking her hand, 'but I know this is the right thing.' She smiled happily. 'We love each other. He's funny and kind, and he treats me really well.' (This was a veiled reference to Polly's ex-boyfriend Harry, a nice but lazy banker, who had been more interested in his bank balance than in Polly.)

'Well I think it's really wonderful,' gushed Kat tossing her head of wild red curls defiantly. This wa unlike the normally shy Kate, who could usually b relied upon for a rather cautious response. Chriss eyed her from head to toe, taking in her smoot honey-coloured skin and her surprisingly svelt toned thighs, revealed to their advantage by h cut-off denims. (At times, Kate had been know to overindulge in the broken rejects from h workplace, Crunch Biscuits.) To top it off, she ha allowed her hair to revert to its naturally curly stat and it was made even prettier by a smattering sun-kissed golden highlights. Chrissie, as reside glamour puss, was not amused.

'It's not like you to be so excitable, Kate. You did have a holiday romance, too, did you?' she purre knowing full well about Kate's unrequited obsessi with her boss, marketing director Matthew.

But Kate remained unruffled, purring back, 'C this isn't about me, Chrissie, this is about P Chrissie bit back her fury – why did she feel so angr

Polly turned to Jaz, who was the only one of h friends who had yet to express an opinion.

'Well, what do you think?' She enquired nervous 'I think you're not taking this seriously enough all,' Jaz responded sternly. 'Don't you realize, Pol she continued, her smile spreading as she caug the look on Polly's crestfallen face, 'that this is t most important dress you're ever going to buy?'

finding a look

rget everything you know about what suits you. hether you live in kitten heels and pretty cardigans or ainers and denim, the chances are that the way you ant to look on your wedding day will be completely related to the way you look in your everyday life. And ery variable will affect the hairstyle that you choose. art by considering the following few elements.

ress style

ave you envisaged yourself in something simple and aty or a huge, structured confection that would be e envy of Cinderella? The way you imagine your dress be and what style actually suits you may be two tirely different things, so take a close friend or family ember shopping with you, and try on lots of different yles. You will be surprised.

ody shape and height

e are all shaped differently, and the satin bias-cut ess of our dreams might not have been part of Mother ature's plan when she made us. As a result, you may ok fabulous enhancing your tiny waist with a fitted dice and hiding your less tiny hips under a full skirt. his means you may need a hairstyle with more body height to create a balanced silhouette.

eckline

ur hairstyle and dress need to work together. A low cooping neckline can look wonderfully romantic with ose tendrils of hair, whereas a chic bob with a sleek ash neck is exceptionally elegant. If you have a low ack on your dress, you can draw attention to this ature by wearing your hair swept up and away from ur neck. Take a photograph or sketch of your dress ith you to the hairdresser's so you can consider which airstyles will make the most of its features.

aras and veils

though it is not uncommon to have both a tiara nd a veil, most brides choose to wear either one

or the other. And, as weddings have become more informal, a few simple flowers dotted through the hair are also a popular alternative to both of these options. A long veil or heavy tiara will need to be held securely in place, and this will influence your choice of hairstyle. If you can, take your tiara (or at least a photograph of it) with you when you go for a consultation with your hairdresser, so that he or she can work out exactly what will need to be done on that count.

face shape

You probably know what suits you by now, and this is not usually the time that women opt for a drastic change of look. (It's nice if he recognizes you when you're walking down the aisle.) However, unless you are a very high-maintenance girl and do your weekly shop wearing a tiara, you probably won't know how it affects the proportions of your face. A petite heart-shaped face may look better with a simple beaded tiara, rather than drowned by a grand crown and full veil. So it's back to dressing up – try on lots of styles and see if your reality matches your fantasy.

jewellery

One of the 'Something old, something new ...' categories is often fulfilled with jewellery. So, whether you choose a string of antique pearls from your grandmother or a funky, dramatic choker from one of your bridesmaids, it needs consideration at this stage, too. A tiara, veil, earrings, choker and high collar can quickly become very fussy. Don't let your look become cluttered – less is always more (even with diamonds).

HAIR SNIP

WHEN CHOOSING ACCESSORIES FOR YOUR HAIR, WHETHER IT IS FRESH FLOWERS OR AN ANTIQUE BROOCH, MAKE SURE IT IS IN BALANCE WITH THE REST OF YOUR OUTFIT – SOMETIMES LESS IS MORE.

In beauty and fashion matters, Jaz is regarded as the oracle, so Polly invites her along to her appointment with her trusted stylist Charles. For the last few years, he has kept her wavy locks blonder and straighter than nature ever intended them to be.

Despite her impetuous decision to get married, Polly's cautious nature has reasserted itself and she pulls from her bag a neat file of pictures from bridal magazines. At the same time, Jaz produces a jumble of catwalk photos, slides from hair shows (borrowed from Aristo PR) and pages torn out of *Gloss* magazine. Charles grins and tells the girls that they need to go back to basics. Polly's hair has a natural wave, which she usually straightens and smooths with a glossing serum. The sun has lightened it to a uniform, creamy blonde that works well with her tan, but makes her fine hair seem thin. They agree that she should have caramel lowlights to make her hair look thicker.

Next, they look at pictures of the dress. Polly has chosen a close-fitting, full-length dress in off-white duchesse satin. Chic and elegant, it has a high neck, three-quarter length sleeves and a low, scooped back. For protection from the elements,

... polly's consultation with charles

she's chosen a fitted high-collar jacket. Charles believes that such a formal dress deserves a formal updo. The hair should be swept up to draw attention to the dramatic plunging dress and show off her slender, tanned back. The next consideration is the jacket, the high collar of which will skim the back of her neck. Charles thinks that to avoid looking fussy, her hairstyle must be simple and clean (which rules out Jaz's pictures of a half-up, half-down do with wispy tendrils and diamanté clips). After much wrangling (veil too much with the jacket, jewellery too fussy for the neckline), they settle on a classic chignon, with a tiara and simple diamond earrings. A slightly despondent Jaz (doesn't Polly know that matrimony is fashionable?) is cheered when Polly escorts her out of the salon telling her it's time to select the bridesmaids' dresses.

condition

e next consideration is the condition of your hair. ead of strong, beautifully conditioned hair will always act the eye (and compliments). You can tackle this ue in two ways – from the inside and the outside.

nside

makes sense that what we put into our bodies l affect how well we look and feel, and the quality ur diet is reflected in the state of our hair. Although can use good-quality shampoos and styling agents enhance the cosmetic appearance of your hair, you improve its condition drastically by giving it the urishment it needs from inside. Hair needs iron, zinc, tein and vitamins A, C and B12. While a good, varied t that includes all of these should be enough for althy hair, a significant deficiency in some of them ch as zinc or vitamin B12) can be linked to hair s. As well as standard vitamin tablets, there are also ecific supplements designed to promote healthy hair, n and nails. Dehydration can have a disastrous effect the condition of the hair, so make sure that you drink east 1.5 litres (2¾ pints) of water every day.

ther important issue for many brides is weight loss. edding extra pounds quickly may be tempting, but if do not diet sensibly you will deprive your hair – and rest of your body – of essential nutrients. When under ess (and crash dieting is an attack on the system), the ly shuts down the delivery of nutrients to all non-ential organs, and first to suffer are the hair and nails. e results of crash dieting can take up to three months show in your hair and will also appear in your skin. n with such an important deadline looming, there is substitute for a sensible exercise and dieting regime.

arning

ou are concerned about a supplement, consult your rmacist. If you experience problems, see your doctor.

Stress, anxiety and sleeplessness can all take their toll on the condition of the hair. Here are a few of the many excellent herbal remedies and supplements that can help:

Calcium and magnesium are often depleted through stress and are needed to help control anxiety and fear.

Camomile tea is soothing and can be great for keeping nerves at bay; it is a good alternative to regular tea, which contains caffeine – a known stimulant that can heighten feelings of anxiety.

Kava kava promotes a feeling of wellbeing and is very good for soothing away tension.

Lavender is a relaxing essential oil. Dilute a few drops in water or vegetable oil and massage it into your scalp. The massage will help increase the blood flow to the scalp and bring nutrients to the hair follicle.

Mimulus helps allay fears over impending events.

Valerian can be used as a relaxant or sleeping aid.

White chestnut stops those constant organizational niggles from keeping you awake at night.

outside

If you have serious concerns, visit a trichologist; hair loss, flaky scalp or dandruff may be signs of a diet deficiency, which can be easily remedied. However, if the bad condition of your hair is due to overprocessing or an ill-advised colour experiment, your hairdresser should be able to help restore your crowning glory. See your hairdresser as soon as possible to give them the opportunity to organize an effective treatment plan. Although treatments have their limitations, a lot can be done to salvage beleaguered hair.

salon solutions

regular trims
Be realistic, and don't skimp on trims just because you want to change your style. If you have only two months until the big day and always imagined having undulating waves to the small of your back, obviously you will have to accept defeat if you are currently sporting a gamine crop (unless you want to go for the full wig option – which is not usually a wise idea if you don't want it to be the topic of conversation all day). Hair grows at an average rate of 1 cm (½ in) per month, and making the classic mistake of scrapping regular trims won't help – split ends will keep on splitting up the hair shaft and look awful. The only permanent remedy is cutting them off.

intense moisture mask
This cream-based conditioning treatment is designed to work on the hair in much the same way as a facial moisturizer works on the skin. Once the cream has been spread evenly through the hair, heat is applied, in the form of hot towels or a dryer, to open the hair shaft and allow the conditioning agents to penetrate the hair shaft fully.

express destress
Tailor-made to tackle your specific hair problems, this treatment often incorporates a scalp and shoulder massage. This helps increase the blood flow (and therefore the delivery of nutrients) to the hair shaft, as well as relieving stress, a serious contributor to dull hair.

intense strengthening mask
Ideal for those who have seriously abused their hair, this liquid-form protein-based moisturizer was designed to give a boost to weak, damaged hair. Your hairdresser may suggest a series of these treatments, as the effects are cumulative. For best results, a glossing conditioner is applied at the final stage.

shine-on colour treatment
Colour is a great way of bringing condition and body to the hair. Even if you are happy with your natural colour, a rinse in the same tone can bring extra gloss and shine. Derived from vegetable extracts, shine-on colours are

excellent for rehydrating dry hair and bringing 'oom back to hair that has already been dyed but has lost original sheen. On fine hair, the colour can plump up hair shaft and add much-needed volume. To prov maximum depth to flat hair, two colours are used, on the top section and one underneath.

It is very important to remember that even so of the gentlest of chemical treatments can dehydr the hair, therefore it might need a little more T than normal. Choose a shampoo, conditioner a styling products that are designed to help maintain yo colour and reduce any discolouring or fading.

scalp energizer
A healthy scalp usually means healthy hair, but e those without scalp problems can benefit from treatment. The exfoliating action leaves the sc exceptionally clean, while the increased blood fl delivers extra nutrients and oxygen to the h improving its condition.

home help
A great way to get your bridesmaids to help with invitations, guest list or any other wedding chore, is have a big girls' night in, under the pretence of so pre-nuptial pampering. You could even make them monthly event, which will do your hair and organizatio skills the world of good.

Most salon treatments can be simplified for home u and there are many great effective treatments availa from your salon or pharmacy. Take a few tips from professionals, and use hot towels and plastic caps encourage the hair shaft to open and to maximize effectiveness of your chosen products.

HAIR S
REMEMBER, ALWAYS RINSE YO
HAIR THOROUGHLY – AND FINISH
WITH AN ICE-COLD RINSE WILL G
MAXIMUM GLOSS AND SHI

ura knows that she has
anged since meeting John,
uch more so than she'd like
 admit. After spending such
ong time hoping to get his
ention, things are moving
etty fast. She's even had to
knowledge that her growing
erest in her appearance is

earlier in the year from a low-
maintenance crop to a slightly
longer fringe (bangs) and light
flick-outs at the nape, is thrilled
to get a second chance to reinvent
Laura. In two and a half months,
hair will grow approximately
2.5 cm (1¼ in). As Laura's
current style is already beginning

to grow out, her stylist suggests
letting the fringe (bangs) grow
out and having it cut over to
one side. The rest of her hair
will be allowed to grow into
a sleek, slightly layered short
bob – feminine, but still right
for Laura's usual uniform of
T-shirt and combats.

.. laura goes for another restyle

ss to do with sharing a flat
th looks-obsessed Chrissie
d Jaz, and more to do with
tching John's attention.

er the initial shock, Laura
s become more supportive
 what she considers to be
lly's impulsive decision to
arry Simon – despite the
ct it might leave them all
meless. It may also have
mething to do with flattery –
lly has asked her to be
aid of Honour (although
ura sometimes wonders
ether Polly reached this
cision largely because of her
ganizational skills, especially
nsidering the lack of help
e's had from the others
th planning the hen night).

ura's decided to see her stylist
out growing her short hair,
ping that a slightly longer style
ll seem less severe next to
lly's sleek updo. Her hairdresser,
ho helped her restyle her hair

wedding
wisdom

As soon as a girl accepts a proposal, everyone has an opinion. Hopefully these tips should help you keep focused on what you want.

1 Start cheating. Don't be despondent if you think your hair doesn't naturally have the qualities you want. This is the most special of occasions and your style doesn't have to be practical or able to function in the real world – just as long as you can make it last the day. There are many tricks of the trade to help you create the illusion that you want: hairpieces can add volume, straighteners can make hair ultra-sleek and a well-placed veil can make even short hair appear long. Your hairdresser could be your greatest ally.

2 If you are wearing a long veil, keep your hairstyle as simple as possible.

3 Don't be tempted to go for a radical restyle – it's you he has asked to marry and it's you he wants to see at the altar.

4 How will you get to the church? Whether it's a horse-drawn carriage or a moped, tell your stylist so that he or she can disaster-proof you!

5 Remember to have long hair trimmed before the big day – even a couple of centimetres (an inch) of growth could make the style you have settled on impossible to achieve.

6 Always have a full trial run with your veil and/or tiara before the big day.

7 If you are not happy with what your hairdresser has done, you must tell them. He or she would rather start again than have it ruin your day.

8 Your dress, veil, flowers, tiara, hair and even shoes should all create a cohesive look – give your stylist as much visual reference as you can to allow them to help you achieve that.

9 There's no need to change hairdressers if you have a good rapport with your current one. He or she knows your hair and how to get the best from it. Do make sure, though, that they feel comfortable doing it. (Your favourite colourist, for example, may not be the person for the job!)

O Don't get an attack of 'wedding ringlets'. If your style is simple, don't let others bully you into a look you don't feel comfortable with just because they perceive it as being more glamorous.

11 Short hair can look just as feminine as longer styles, and if you know that it suits you, you're better off sticking with what you've got.

2 Some subtle highlights around the face are a great way to lift the complexion and draw attention to the face.

13 Make sure you give plenty of notice if you want a particular stylist to do your hair on the morning of the wedding.

4 Using every styling product on the market to and keep your hair in place will only make it look ty and weighed down. Select products well and ve a trial run to see how much you really need.

15 Work with your hair type if you can – will your long, poker-straight hair really stay in curls all day?

16 Take a camera to the hairdresser's with you. You will be surprised how something that looks good in real life doesn't always look great in photographs. This will also give you some reference material to show to your family and friends.

17 You must start planning your hairstyle approximately three months in advance. This means that you will have the time to get your hair into top condition, with two or three conditioning treatments at your salon, and have two trial runs of the actual style. Having trial runs will make sure you get the style just right so that you feel more positive about the day.

countdown

In an ideal world, brides would begin thinking about their haircare regime at least nine months before the wedding. This would allow ample time to improve the condition of the hair with treatments and any necessary changes to diet and lifestyle before even choosing a hairstyle. This is especially important if you suffer from alopecia (hair loss) or seborheic dermatitis (a condition that results in a flaky scalp); these are often caused by a dietry deficiency and can be treated by a trichologist (see page 239). Likewise, if your hair is in poor condition due to chemical processing or overstyling, make an appointment to see your hairdresser as soon as you can to allow time for them to implement an effective treatment programme.

Ultimately, your hairdo and the accessories you choose should reflect your style and personality in the same way as your choice of dress. So, while it is a good idea to gather inspiration from magazines, don't force yourself to adopt a look that is not really 'you'. Try not to change yourself too much, but make the most of what you've got and maximize your good points. Always take a photo or sketch of your dress and a swatch of fabric to your first hair consultation and ask your hairdresser's advice on accessories and flowers. You might like to try out a few different hairstyles before settling on the right one, and always have a full trial run – complete with accessories, veil and tiara – in advance of the big day. Take someone with you whose advice you trust for an honest second opinion. Use the table below to help you plan ahead.

pre-wedding hair tip

Are you using the right haircare products for yo hair type? For example, if your hair is fine and la this may be due to your conditioner being t heavy. Assess the condition of your hair and lo at your current haircare regim

Collect pictures for your scrapbook of hairsty and colours that you like from all sources, not ju from wedding magazin

Do take polaroids of your hair rehearsals – otherw it will be impossible for you or your hairdresser remember every det

Even if results seem slow to emerge, stick w your treatment plan. The effects are cumulat and the end result will be worth

In the period leading up to your wedding, try a give your hair a break from intensive styl methods whenever possib

Florists can provide blooms all year round no but find out which will be in season on the big d It's a sweet reminder of your wedding to see flowers you wore in your hair in bloom for yo anniversary in years to con

6 months	5 months	4 months	3 months	2 months	1 month
See your hair-dresser to discuss your plans and book in all your appointments.	Experiment with various colour options so you can achieve the optimum look.	Collect a scrapbook of style options and discuss these with your stylist.	Begin weekly conditioning treatments.	Order the flowers for your hair. Have your first trial run at the salon.	Have a secon trial run with your veil/tiara Reconfirm your final cut and colour.

get the look

wedding fever hits the house

Every surface of Polly's formerly immaculate house was covered with wedding magazines, invitations, lists and scraps of fabric.

'I would have thought,' said Chrissie, pinching a piece of Laura's toast and munching it cautiously through her regular Saturday morning face pack, 'that you would have approached this wedding with your usual degree of organization.' Laura and Kate exchanged glances. Chrissie was becoming unbearable, always ready with a sharp word or criticism.

'You try organizing a wedding in only two months,' sighed Polly, oblivious of Chrissie's critical tone. 'Now, let's get on with the business in hand – your outfits.'

Jaz started to wriggle on her chair, never more excited than when talking about clothes. 'Well, girls, we chose the fabric last week and I think you are just going to love it!' she squealed. The girls held their breath collectively – why on earth was Polly letting Jaz choose their dresses? Did she really want them tripping down the aisle in leopard skin and neon fishnets? Jaz pulled out two swatches of fabric, silk georgette in pale pink and lilac. So far, so elegant. Surely there had to be a catch.

'We thought,' said Polly, enjoying their surprise, 'or rather Jaz did, that these two colours would suit all your hair and skin tones.'

'And,' added Jaz excitedly, 'that we would have each dress in the colour you choose with a contrasting detail. For example, Laura, with your dark hair, you'd look lovely in lilac with a spilt revealing the pink; and Kate, you'd suit pink with a draped neck lined with lilac.'

Chrissie was impressed and slightly annoyed – maybe Jaz knew more about fashion than just trends. 'So we don't all have to look the same?' she asked – she hated the thought of resembling anyone else.

'Well, within reason,' cautioned Polly. 'But since you're all different shapes, as well as such different characters, it makes sense to let you all have an input and make the most of your best features.'

'And what about our hair?' asked Chrissie, who had long believed that her straight, blonde, shiny h was the secret to all her powers. She had be praying that Polly wouldn't expect her to hide it away in a childish corn plait or, worse, an attack dreaded 'wedding ringlets'.

'Well, I want you all to incorporate some little p roses into your style in some way, but how entirely up to you. Just nothing too crazy,' P said, eyeing Jaz's latest tie-dyed style.

'What about your hair?' asked Kate. Polly beame 'Well, I'm not giving too much away, but I saw Char last week and we have a plan – I'm getting it cut a coloured the week before, and in the mean time h having treatments every two weeks to improve t condition.' She paused to pop a slab of buttery, wh muffin into her mouth. Kate looked startled.

'But don't you know that what you put into yo body is just as influential to your hair's condition what you treat it with externally? By the time you g married all the stress of the planning, late nigh and takeaways will start showing in your hair.' Po sipped her coffee guiltily – Kate was right, she ha been pushing herself extra hard at work to get thin finished so she could go on a long honeymoon. Sim was still in New York, so all the planning was le mainly to her. On top of that, she still hadn't told t girls that she wasn't moving to New York to be wi Simon, but that he would be transferring to Londo That meant that they would want the house f themselves – and the girls would have to move ou She was definitely a woman under pressure.

'There's nothing like a convert for giving unsolicit advice,' said Chrissie, referring to Kate's rece transformation from biscuit-muncher to abs-crunche Sensing Kate's and Chrissie's rivalry, Laura stepped i 'Don't forget, everyone, that I expect you all to b ready to hit the bars running next Saturday for on of Polly's last nights of freedom.' She wrapped a arm around each of the girls' shoulders, 'and expect all of Polly's friends to be very friendly.'

boho vintage

This girl is never happier than when rummaging through antique shops and flea markets, searching for vintage tea dresses, silk gloves and beaded purses. At the end of her bed she keeps an old pine trunk, overflowing with diaphanous slips, pretty scraps of antique lace and crochet, and romantic Victorian nightgowns. For her wedding day, she'd team a snugly fitting Edwardian bodice with a full tulle skirt, and wear a romantic amethyst choker at her throat.

hair solutions

If you have long hair, you cou opt for a half-up, half-down o with your hair half obscuring yo crown, but with delicate tendr framing your face. Mid-length ha can create the illusion of leng when it is pulled back under a tw tier lace veil. Short hair can softened with light-hold wax ar decorated with beaded clips ornaments, such as butterflies.

LEFT AND RIGHT

The hair is tonged using a light blow-dry spray to give flexibility and movement. Three bun rings are pinned together and placed on the crown of the head. The hair is wrapped around the rings, pinned securely in place and finished with firm-hold hairspray. A natural-coloured cord is wound around the hair and fastened behind the ear. If you want to dress the hair further, add an ornate hair pin on one side of the head, and hold it in place using fine pins.

OVERLEAF

To create this romantic look, you can employ either the classic technique of plaiting damp hair and leaving it to dry before you unravel the plaits, or the modern technique of using a hot waving iron. Use a glossing spray to finish and simply dress the style with a fine necklace or hair ornament pinned around the forehead.

country

The girl who goes for the country style loves all things pretty and natural, and that includes her look. Her dress will be a simple, feminine home-made affair; she'll carry a bouquet of wild flowers and wear a garland in her hair.

hair solutions

Keep your hair unstructured and, if it's long, flowing loose over your shoulders. Flowers are the obvious choice for decoration, but keep them simple, small and dotted throughout the hair. Alternatively, take two sections of hair from the front and plait them, incorporating fine ribbons in shades of bright and baby pink; secure the back with a band and conceal it by wrapping a length of ribbon around it. A wild flower garland creates a feminine look for short hair.

BELOW AND RIGHT

The hair is sectioned into narrow segments, working forwards from the centre of the crown, twisted into tight knots and secured along the hairline with mat grips. The ends of the hair are left loose for a natura romantic finish. For a dramatic look, decorate the knots with feathers that match your outfit.

OVERLEAF

Sections of the hair are sprayed using a fine-hold hairspray, and various sizes of tongs are used to create romantic ringlets. These can be left *au natu* for a stronger look (left), or the curls can be broke up with fingers for a Lady Godiva look (right). Finis with gloss or serum to add curl definition. Various accessories can be used – from natural blooms to tiaras and strands of diamanté beads.

own up?' exclaims Jaz's
list, Zoe. She's been doing
z's hair since she was a junior
list and has tried out all of
most directional looks on her.
nods firmly. Her job at Astrid
is everything she had hoped
vould be, but she's started to
nk that she's being overlooked
promotion. Her cutting-edge
k is great when she's dealing
h designers or at the shows,
when it comes to important
etings she's often left behind.
it because Astrid feels she
n't deal with the business side
things? Or just that she can't
them to take her seriously in
present incarnation? Either
y, she's ready for a change.

ant to go for a classic, straight
p with a blunt fringe [bangs],'
ys Jaz. Zoe raises an eyebrow.
a, the power bob. Trouble at
rk?' she asks. 'First of all, Jaz,
need to look like you, and
t is so not your style. Secondly,
vill drown your face. just look

... jaz goes for a grown-up look

your face shape.' Zoe is right;
z's slim heart-shaped face
uldn't carry off such a look.
hy don't we meet halfway?'
e suggests, 'and dye it back to
natural black, then cut it into
ong bob, sloping down at the
nt and without a fringe. If we
or the ends, you can stop it
m hanging in a single, heavy
unk. That way you have lots of
rsatility when you're not being
s Business Woman.'

'Sounds like you and I are changing
places,' giggles Kate, slipping
into the chair next to Jaz.
'Kate! What are you doing here?'
asks Jaz, slightly unnerved to be
caught dicing with conformity.
'I'm getting back to my roots,
literally,' says Kate. 'My highlights
from the holiday are growing out,
so I'm having a vegetable colour
put on to bring back my normal
titian colour.' Jaz eyes her old
school friend in the mirror. She

looks great; she hasn't used
her hair straighteners since her
return, letting her natural curl
reassert itself with a vengeance.
She seems so much more
confident and relaxed than
the girl who went away.
'Is there something you're not
telling me?' Jaz enquires. Kate
smiles as Zoe leads Jaz away
to wash her hair.
'No,' she says. 'It's just that some
things are better left unspoilt.'

urbanite

Everything in her life is luxurious but with a thoroughly modern edge. She's a high-maintenance girl whose wardrobe is filled with elegant, well-cut clothes and whose look is one of understated glamour. Naturally, her wedding outfit is no exception. She'll be wearing an exquisitely cut white trouser suit with a plunging neckline revealing a fair amount of bare *décolletage*. Jewellery will be simple and modern, and a flower-ball bouquet will be dangling from her slender wrist.

hair solutions

Short hair naturally complem this sharp look, while mid-ler hair is best in a 1920s-style Long hair is great poker-stra with an extreme side parting ar section pulled back into a fea headdress. Keep it simple, with accent on impeccable condition.

LEFT AND RIGHT

For the textured look (right), th hair is tousled using wet-look g to give a glossy, almost glass-li finish. The hair on the crown is st using the fingers to give textu height and a spiky finish. If you h short hair but want a longer lc use a ¾ hairpiece to add lengt and interest around the face (lef

OVERLEAF LEFT

The hair is scrunch-dried using blow-dry primer spray for volur and texture. It is swept back in high ponytail, and backbrushed sculpted into the required shap The style is finished with a firm-h hairspray and a necklace or brac pinned to the front of the 'sculptu A veil-type fringe is also an opti

OVERLEAF RIGHT

The hair is slicked back into a m height ponytail and set on heat rollers. The curls are broken uf with the fingers and piled into a clear, natural hairnet, secured wi fine pins. A feathered comb ca be added to the side of the bur

audrey

Her biggest style influence is, of course, Audrey Hepburn in *Breakfast at Tiffany's*. She always looks well groomed and classically elegant – her uniform is crisp linen shift dresses for summer and neat pencil skirts and fitted sweaters for winter. For her wedding, she'll be wearing a sleeveless column dress in off-white satin, and carrying either a tight posy of cream roses tied with pale blue ribbon or a single long-stemmed amaryllis or lily.

hair solutions

Smoothing your long hair into neat chignon, with a subtle tia and a satin-trimmed shoulde length veil, is a perfectly class look. Mid-length hair looks gre accessorized with an Alice ba and mini-veil, while vivid orchids a green tendrils secured behind o ear are ideal for short hair.

LEFT

The hair is set on medium-sized rollers using a fine flexi-hold hair-spray and allowed to cool totally before gently removing them. The curls are broken up using a large toothed comb and the root area of the crown is backcombed. The sides are smoothed back and pinned with matt grips. A decorativ comb completes the look.

RIGHT

The hair is swept up into a neat high ponytail in the centre of the head. It is then set on heated rollers, which are removed when they are totally cool. The hair is pulled through two bun rings over which the curls are placed and pinned. A necklace can be pinned across the hairline for decoration.

HAIR SN

BALANCE IS ABSOLUTELY ESSENTIA
DO NOT GO TOO BIG IF YOU AF
TALL, BUT TRY BIGGER HAIR IF YC
ARE ON THE SHORT SIDE – YO
NEVER KNOW, YOU MAY LOVE

classic

'Refined good taste' are this girl's watchwords. She always looks immaculate, even on casual days. For work she wears beautifully tailored suits and relaxes at the weekend in smart but fashionable denim or cords. She thrives on tradition and ceremony, and never more so than at her own wedding. Her elegant empire-line gown in duchesse satin is offset with a frothy white veil and a trailing bouquet of white flowers and green foliage for a timelessly stylish look.

hair solutions

This is perfect for those who want the quintessential bridal look of veil and tiara. A crown tiara is great on short hair, while long hair demands to be piled up high. For fine or mid length hair, try adding a hairpiece.

LEFT AND RIGHT

Ultra-glossy hair is swept back and secured into a French pleat using fine pins and matt grips. A small circular tiara is placed onto the crown, and a plaited section of hair is positioned inside and held in place with hair pins and hairspray.

OVERLEAF LEFT

The root area of freshly blow-dried or set hair is backbrushed. The nape section is swept up to the crown and secured with matt grips. The top section is brought over, wound down onto the mid-section and fastened with matt grips to create a soft roll. Accessories or feathers can be added to the base of the roll.

OVERLEAF RIGHT

The hair is set on medium-sized rollers using a fine flexi-hold hair-spray. When cool, the rollers are removed and the curls are broken up using a large-toothed comb. Using fingers as a comb, the hair is shaped around the face in large sweeping waves. For gentle hold, hairspray is applied to the fingers and run through the hair.

rock chick

This girl loves to play – and her wedding day will be no exception. Her usual uniform is skin-tight denim, tiny ripped T-shirts, leather cuffs and high-heeled snake-skin ankle boots. Her bridal version will comprise a very short skirt, a slash-neck top and fishnets – all in snowy white. She won't carry flowers, but will finish off the look with a diamanté collar and cuffs, smoky eyes and hair with serious attitude.

hair solutions

Regardless of length, the look he is big, big, big. Lots of texture a backcombing will give long hair th super-sexy just-about-to-fall-int bed-head look – but remember use products only at the roots, or t hair will be weighed down. Wi shorter hair, try a tiara on a chopp textured cut. On any length, dor forget height at the crown.

LEFT AND RIGHT

For a classic rock-chick look, the hair is dyed 'peroxide' blonde and cut dry using a razor to inject some attitude into this modern style. Wax is used to give a matt, chunky finish and a sparkling crystal tiara makes this look a little more feminine.

OVERLEAF LEFT

For an ultra-modern rock-chick look, the hair is cut randomly using texturizing scissors and coloured with a variety of red and petrol tones to create an edgy effect.

OVERLEAF RIGHT

The hair is blow-dried using blow-dry priming spray to give volume and create a tendril effect. It is then pulled up into ponytails along the centre of the head in a mohican formation, then randomly placed and pinned to give a soft but edgy finish. Fake hairpieces can be added for extra drama if desired.

fashionista

Luckily, marriage is back in fashion and this bride-to-be has embraced it with as much enthusiasm as she always has for designer sales. Her dress will be *couture*, of course – a bright pink slip covered with transparent, spider-web lace. She'll be sashaying down the aisle as though it were a catwalk, wearing perilously high strappy slingbacks. Flowers are a wrist corsage or choker, consisting of a single orchid.

hair solutions

Whatever the length of your ha its condition is vital, so make su you book in for some conditionir treatments well before the big da On long hair, instead wearing a traditional tiara, try pinning necklace across the forehead ov unstructured big hair. A short style can look stunning when t hair is textured and single diaman studs are clipped into it. Mediur length hair looks feminine in shaggy style – create the separati by twisting damp, moussed hair ir bands and leaving it to dry. Bead flower clips can be used to pull ha back and draw attention to the fac

LEFT

This is achieved with a 'scrumpling technique, which provides a modern take on curly hair. The hair is drenched with mousse, scrumpled down and pinned, ther left to dry. The pins are removed and the hair is formed and shape into the required style. A firm-hol hairspray sets and holds the styl Add a modern band or tiara to maximize the dramatic impact.

RIGHT

The hair is swept back into a twist, leaving the ends to splay out to one side of the head in a fan effect. Wax is used to give definition and texture to the end A theatrical necklace works well as a modern skull-cap.

It's **Saturday night** and the girls are rushing around, brushes in hand, music blaring and empty wine bottles starting to gather on the kitchen table.

'Oh god, I look like a sheepdog,' moans Laura, trying to tease her hair, which has reached the highly unpopular 'difficult' stage, into some kind of style. Jaz pops her hair around the bathroom door.

'Want some help?' she offers, looking as if she's never had a bad-hair day in her life. She loves her new style so much that she's left it hanging loose, dressing it up with only a slick of blue hair mascara to enhance the natural glossy blackness. Luckily, her dressing table is still littered with every beauty fix and whimsy on the market. She grabs some

hair grips with subtle flowers fashioned from jade and ruby beads. Laura looks dubious as Jaz runs a little texturizing wax through her hair, pulling the shorter sections from the front and twisting them into ridges. Despite Laura's general aversion to all things feminine, she has to admit that Jaz has made a virtue of her hair's unruliness.

... the girls get ready to party

Chrissie limps past with one foot in a tiger-print mule, and spies the missing one poking out from underneath Jaz's bed. Remembering Laura's warning, she bites back her annoyance, only to catch a glimpse of Laura looking fabulous in casual jeans with her hair in a pretty half-updo. Determined not to be outdone by the house tomboy, she stomps back into her room to turn her plaits into something a bit more glamorous.

Chrissie flicks through *Gloss* magazine until she finds a picture of her favourite glam 'do' of the moment – the 1970s-inspired flick. She applies some volumizing mousse to the front section of her long hair, and then winds it around a huge Velcro roller. After a blast of hot air from her hairdryer and a spritz of hairspray, she leaves it to set and gets to work with the lip gloss.

romantic

This girl is a true romantic. She loves nothing better than watching reruns of *Gone with the Wind* on rainy days – and it never fails to bring tears to her eyes. She's been planning her wedding day for as long as she can remember. Her dress will be fit for a princess – a beautiful full-skirted, tight-bodiced affair with the longest train she can find – and there will be flowers everywhere, in blushing pink and cream.

hair solutions

Long hair will be worn loose a full with a gentle wave and fre flowers woven into it at the crow With mid-length hair, fresh t roses in muted purples and pin can be used to form a natur Alice band over the crown. You c create a dramatic short-hair lo by smoothing hair away from t face with a beaded tiara.

LEFT AND RIGHT

This is a very modern take on the classic pin curl. Sections of hair, approximately 5 cm (2 in) square are twisted around the fingers and pinned in place all over the head using matt hair grips. Large fresh flowers are interspersed between the curls.

OVERLEAF

Very straight, long hair is tonged using large-barrelled hot tongs to create gentle waves that are left loose to cascade down the back. For added interest a natural flower garland is pinned in place in the centre of the crown.

HAIR SN

IF YOU ARE USING FRESH FLOWEF IN YOUR HAIR, CAREFULLY SPRI THEM WITH WATER USING A VEF FINE SPRAY TO PREVENT THE FROM DROOPING AND KEE THEM FRESH ALL DAY LON

beach

This fun- and sun-loving girl is the ultimate beach babe, so it's no surprise that she wants a wedding by the sea. She'll wear a strappy white dress or a string bikini and toe rings, with only her parasol to shield her from the rays.

hair solutions

Minimum fuss with maximum effect is the order of the day here. Whatever your hair length, running some hair oil through your locks will keep it protected from the sun and sea air. Long hair looks great secured in a low bun off to one side at the nape of the neck. Pull some loose ends out to keep it playful. Veils and tiaras are pretty much out, but a big, exotic single bloom can look great tucked behind your ear.

LEFT AND BELOW LEFT

The hair is tonged using multi-sized barrelled tongs to give loose romantic ringlets. An anti-humidity blow-dry spray is used to maximize the longevity of the style and also to minimize frizz. Alternatively, the curls can be broken up with a light serum and a comb pulled through the top section and secured above the crown (below left).

BELOW

The hair is sectioned into 2.5-cm (1-in) squares. Ribbons, chosen to match the outfit, are tied around the base of each section of hair and then wrapped around its length in a crisscross formation, keeping the tension all the way down, and tied securely at the ends of the hair. The ends of the ribbons can either be left to hang free, or snipped off for a tidier look.

the big day

the big day dawns at last ...

'You are so sly!' giggled Polly, as she accepted a glass of Champagne from Kate. Kate had finally let everyone in on her news – which explained her recent secrecy and absences from the house.

'Well, I wanted to make sure that I'd been accepted before I told you,' she said. 'And also, the course I want to do, the only one that combines nutrition and physiotherapy, is based in Edinburgh ... which means I'll be moving out.' Polly looked up from under the slab of backcombed fringe (bangs) that currently flopped in front of her face.

'I'm glad you've brought that up,' she began, 'because there's something I have to tell you all, too. We've decided to live in London. It'll take at least three months to organize Simon's transfer, so there's plenty of time to make other arrangements.' She looked imploringly at each of her friends.

'Oh, stop looking like Bambi,' said Chrissie. 'We're all big girls, you know, we'll be fine!' Laura nodded in agreement, but secretly wasn't so sure. Things between her and John had been strained recently, and she was concerned that maybe he was starting to go off her. Instead of chatting and laughing away as usual, he seemed withdrawn and anxious.

'Polly, unless you to want to wear your crown around your neck it might be a good idea to keep your head still,' chided Charles affectionately. He had come to Polly's home as a special treat for her big day. Keeping her silky, fine blonde hair in a chignon was going to take all his skill and a few industry tricks. He began by applying thickening spray to the hair and winding it onto large rollers to give as much height and body as possible. After drying the hair,

he gave it a burst of hot then cold air to help h[ ] the shape, and then removed the rollers. Char[ ] then scooped back the hair into a classic tw[ ] and attached the tiara, a delicate pearl affa[ ] towards the front of the crown. After a fine spr[ ] of firm-hold hairspray, Charles stepped back [ ] admire his work. It was the perfect look for Po[ ] elegant and simple but with enough grandeur [ ] carry off her glamorous gown.

Despite her original concerns about allowing t[ ] girls to choose their own dresses and hairstyl[ ] they all looked fantastic. Jaz had chosen a p[ ] dress, tied on one shoulder with an asymmetri[ ] hem. Her sleek black hair followed her hemli[ ] parted to one side and secured with a cluster of p[ ] roses attached to a sequinned clip. She also wor[ ] wrist band of roses. Polly had never seen Lau[ ] looking as feminine as she did in her long lilac sh[ ] dress with a low, draped back, her hair in a sh[ ] bob with a band of pale pink roses against her d[ ] hair. Kate had left her hair loose, with roses dott[ ] through its tumbling curls. Her milky complexion w[ ] set off perfectly against the pink of her knee-leng[ ] dress, which, as Jaz had advised had a sligh[ ] draped neck. Chrissie, whose natural instinct w[ ] to grab attention wherever she could, had chos[ ] a flowing style in pink, with contrasting lilac ruff[ ] and a split starting at mid-thigh. A large rose w[ ] pinned behind one ear, pulling back her full blon[ ] hair. The dress had caused Laura to scowl wh[ ] Chrissie had pulled it off the hanger, but Polly lov[ ] it. It was exactly what she would have expected, an[ ] was their differences that she loved them for.

on the day

...e to all your hard work and preparation, your hair ...uld now be in fabulous condition, ready and waiting to ...transformed into your chosen style. Resist the urge ...slather on conditioner for a last-minute boost, or fill ...r hair with extra product – it will only weigh it down. ...ck to your tried-and-tested routine.

...entourage

...he same way that you wouldn't leave your bridesmaids' ...sses until the last minute, you should also consider in ...rance how their hairstyles will work with yours. Are you ...ming your looks and want them to have scaled-down ...sions of your style? Is this practical? Will they feel ...re comfortable in a style similar to their normal look?

...ey thing to consider is the ages of your bridesmaids. ...tle girls are usually happy to take instruction, but ...ult bridesmaids will often have strong feelings about ...eir look. It is sometimes better (and more harmonious) ...bridesmaids are allowed to wear their hair – and ...sses – in a more individual way (it is also highly ...ikely that grown-up bridesmaids will have similar ...rstyles). A great way to do this is by using flowers, ...all tiaras or hair accessories and allowing them ...be interpreted in individual ways. Try to create an ...mosphere that will allow your bridesmaids to tell you ...hey are uncomfortable. Ask them to keep a scrapbook ...looks they like and see if you can find a compromise.

...roducts

...hough there is a whole array of hair products ...ailable to help you achieve your perfect look, they will ...most effective if you use fewer of them in the right ...mbination. Remember, the products you use every ...y may not be right for achieving a more elaborate ...rstyle, so make sure you select the right ones.

mousse

This airy foam will thicken flyaway hair and give control with a natural appearance.

curl activator

Curly hair can sometimes suffer from lack of moisture, which this product is packed full of. Use it sparingly, though, as too much can turn definition into wet-look.

gel

Ideal for controlling and volumizing short or fine hair, gel is a bride's best friend. Even if you've never used if before, consider using it for updos and to tame unruly wisps.

hairspray

The classic mistake for those needing staying power is to spray too much of this stylist's staple, rather than selecting the right holding strength. This will give your hair a hard look and dull its shine. Get the strength right in the first place and it will last.

styling crème

Some leave-in conditioners also double as a styling crème, which can create a smooth, flat finish. It can also be used on dry ends. Use it sparingly.

serum

This can be used to control frizz or enhance shine. It is a great way to make the hair look healthily polished, but don't use too much, as it can make the hair look greasy.

wax and pomade

These range from a hard, shoe polish-like wax to a softer, creamy texture. Use these products to create excellent definition on short hair, and to separate strands and enhance the layers of long hair or a fringe (bangs).

shine spray

Similar to serum, this can be used on top of other products to restore gloss.

Ceremony over, guests greeted and speeches read, Polly slips away to spice up her look for the evening reception, taking the girls for company.

'I hope Simon's parents will recognize you when you return,' giggles Laura, as Jaz produces powders and potions from her seemingly bottomless bag.

'Not that it matters,' says Kate. 'Now that you're Mrs Simon they can hardly call off the wedding.' Polly smiles serenely. Everything had been perfect. It had been a wonderful Indian-summer day; all of the people she loves had been around her, and watching Simon waiting for her at the top of the aisle had given her the best feeling she'd ever known.

'Can you turn into the light a bit Pol?' asks Jaz, removing Polly's tiara and unpinning her chignon as Charles had shown her. She takes a large bristle brush and brushes out the hairspray, letting the hair bounce back in big, soft curls. Grabbing some styling spray from the SOS kit, she sprays Polly's upturned head to help maintain body. Jaz smooths back the top front section, and holds it in place with a crystal beaded slide, creating a 1950s inspired half-up, half-down style

... polly's day-to-night transformation

'Don't go too crazy with the gold look,' Polly warns Jaz, who had promised to create a spectacular night-time look for her. In moments of pre-wedding anxiety she had imagined leading the first dance with glittery striped cheekbones. 'You lot have such little faith in me,' says Jaz, slipping a glitter stick back into her make-up bag. 'When have I ever been Over The Top?' The girls cackle wildly as they remind each other of Jaz' more extreme forays into fashion – her tie-dyed hair, her luminous fishnet tights ... Jaz just smiles and begins dusting shimmering gold powder on Polly's cheekbones and hair. After an extra layer of mascara and a touch of eyeliner to enhance Polly's blue eyes, she slicks some clear gloss across her lips, a look that's glamorous without being heavy. 'OK, you comedians,' she says standing back to admire her handy work. 'It's time to get Mrs Simon back to her party.'

making it last

Whether you are doing your own wedding hair or visiting your stylist, there are certain tricks that will give your hair extra staying power. Make sure your bridesmaids and mother read these tips, too!

1 If you are having an updo, wash your hair the night before the wedding, rather than on the day, since just-washed hair can be harder to tame. Those with a fringe (bangs) may want to part the front section and wash that separately.

2 When you use any styling product, it is very important that most of it is applied at the roots, not the ends. This will stop the hair from being too flat.

3 Silky hair that usually hangs loose in a pretty but stubborn curtain can be tamed by the addition of styling agents. Thickening volumizing spray, wax and mousse will all help the tiara or veil grip onto the hair. Make sure that you do not overcondition fine hair, as this will weigh it down.

4 To put more volume into your style, alternate between hot and cold heat settings when you are blow-drying your hair. Dry the hair first using hot air, then give each section a cold blast – this will set in body and bounce as the hair cools down and will help to hold the style in shape for longer.

5 Extra-large rollers will create great volume. Work from the top to the bottom of the head, taking sections of hair that are approximately 2.5–5 cm (1–2 in) wide, depending on its length and health. Roll the hair under in the direction you want the style to lay and ensure that the rollers sit snugly against the scalp for maximum body. Once all the rollers have been inserted, spritz the hair with a styling spray for long-lasting root lift.

6 Roller-set your hair to make it more manageable and easier to put up on the day.

7 When using hair products, try to choose them all from the same range for the most effective result – they are designed to work together.

8 Backcombing is the backbone of all updos, giving both volume and staying pow It may look bad for your hair but it is essent

Having a trial run with your veil and tiara is extrem important. Clear combs are the most effective way securing a veil discreetly and firmly, and you may ne to employ matt grips in a shade similar to your h colour for extra support. Tiaras often come with hoc for slides to be slipped into or with a comb to grip hair as part of their design. Give your style a serio workout to make sure it has staying power; you v be miserable if you find yourself anxiously trying balance a slipping tiara all day. Backcombing of helps give the hair texture to which things can grip, will using product in the hair. Always ask the st from which you buy your veil or tiara to show you h to secure it – they are the experts.

SOS kit

No bride should venture into the elements without her S kit. Take whatever you need to feel secure, then nomin your bridesmaid with the biggest handbag to look after

Hairspray and shine spray
Matt hair grips and hair pins – and plenty of them
Natural-bristle smoothing brush
Tail comb
Hot rollers
Bun ring
Hairpiece

can't believe I'm doing this,' utters Chrissie, as she prepares to dash out into the rain to collect Polly's bag from the car. The weather has finally broken, the clear skies turning black with heavy showers. After five minutes in the doorway of the country hotel where the reception is being held, she finally accepts that she'll just have to make a run for it.

The 20-second round trip leaves her completely soaked. Her hair is plastered to her head and her lovely dress is glued to her skin. As she slinks through the door, hugging the wall, and starts up the stairs to the suite, she spots Knell Kendrew, the head of Devastation Records arriving at the reception. She could weep on the spot. Never one to indulge in soul-searching, Chrissie's finally realized what

... chrissie gets caught in the rain

has been making her so touchy of late. It seems that everyone else is moving on in their lives, while she's left stuck behind the reception desk at Devastation Records, waiting for the big break that never seems to come.

'There you are! You're soaked and it's completely my fault!' cries Polly, making her way down the stairs towards her, in her freshly made-up perfection.

'Don't panic anyone,' says Jaz, rummaging in her bag with one hand and nudging Chrissie into the suite with the other. 'Charles left me an SOS kit for exactly this kind of crisis. Get that dress off.'

Once inside, Chrissie wriggles out of her wet dress, drapes it on the radiator and shrugs on one of the fluffy white dressing gowns hanging on the door. She takes a seat at the dressing

table and begins removing her melting mascara. Jaz combs some shine spray from Charles's SOS kit through the length of Chrissie's hair. With some deft twisting, she pulls it back into a band, folds the hair over and secures it into a low, loose bun, with a few strands pulled out. The effect is pretty and sexy – the perfect match for her ruffled dress. Maybe she isn't going to have to hide from Knell after all.

post-ceremony

Once the ceremony is over, a grand style may seem slightly extreme, so perform a quick transformation by detaching your veil and leaving your tiara in place.

day to night

For a different evening look, make sure your daytime style can translate easily into night-time glamour. Too much product will leave the hair lank and dull, so use one that will brush out easily, such as hairspray. Take a bridesmaid with you when trying out looks with your hairdresser so that she can see how your style needs to be changed, using your own SOS kit.

LEFT
The hair is divided into 2.5-cm (1-in) square sections, and each one is bound with thin copper

wire which allows you to sculpt the tendrils into the desired shape. Finish off with a simple accessory

going away

If you are travelling as soon as the reception is over, you'll want a hairstyle that is tidy and manageable. If you have long hair, try a chic, simple ponytail or scooped-chignon, while a smudge of wax is great for tousling slicking back short hair. Some wedding-day hairstyles are likely to leave your hair kinky and unmanageable when you remove all the grips and paraphernalia. Happily, this means that you can employ the classic going-away style – the Grace Kelly headscarf.

RIGHT
For this glamorous 'Jackie O' look, the hair is set on large heated rollers to give volume and wave, and then backcombed at the roots to create big-impact hair. Finish off with a spritz of hairspray to hold.

post-ceremony hair tips

Plan your day-to-night and going-away styles before the day. You may need to buy extra kit

If your wedding-day hairstyle looks fine with your going-away outfit, don't change it for the sake of

Keep it simple – by the time you leave the reception you won't want to fuss over something complicated

Don't be tempted to add lots more extra product it will only make your hair look limp and dull

Make sure you can travel with your hairstyle – you don't want to have to sit bolt upright on a long flight

Take your SOS kit with you in your hand luggage

happily ever after ...

All of the girls, except Chrissie, were hovering in the doorway of the plush country hotel, waiting for the happy couple to make their exit.

'Well, I think we should move to East London. That's where everything happens these days; don't you think so, Laura?' said Jaz. Laura mumbled non-commitally. She had hoped that maybe she wouldn't be sharing a house anymore – at least, not with her girlfriends. But judging from John's mood this evening, he seemed less likely to want to co-habit than inhabit another country altogether.

'Oh, look!' cried Kate, breaking her train of thought, 'Here they come!' Kisses, tears, hugs and more confetti rained down on the wedding party as the couple slowly made their way through the crowd. Jaz looked around frantically, 'Where is Chrissie? She's going to miss them!' On cue, Chrissie came bobbing through the crowd. An arm reached out and pulled her out of the throng. It was Knell.

'Chrissie?' she said. Chrissie looked up at Knell, the most powerful woman at Devastation Records, and smiled nervously. She was unsure how to respond to the older woman, knowing that her looks and flirty charms would have no effect.

'Oh, hi Knell, what are you doing here?' she managed to ask.

'Simon's good friends with my son,' Knell explained. 'They were at university together in the States. Anyway, I'm glad to have bumped into you here, I've seen a different side to you this evening.'

'Yeah, I bet you have,' thought Chrissie gloomily. Herself wearing a wrinkled dress and her make-up washed off by a torrential downpour was not the kind of lasting impression she wanted to linger with Knell. 'I suppose you wondered why you didn't get the gig with Pout,' Knell continued, referring to Chrissie unsuccessful audition for a girl band earlier in th year. 'It was because you didn't bring anything ne and different. Basically, you were the same as th girls already in the band – all polish and perfectior Chrissie winced internally, reminded of why Kne was regarded as one of the toughest women in th industry. Knell placed an arm around her shoulder 'But seeing you tonight has made me reconside Maybe what you need is a change of image something more natural. People are growing tire of the same old manufactured girl-band line-up Come and see me on Monday, we'll talk.' Knell gent pushed Chrissie back into the crowd, signifying tha their meeting was over. Chrissie continued he struggle to get to the girls in a state of shock. Mayb she was going to get her shot at the limelight after a and, even better, she wasn't going to have to share

'Quick, here they come,' squealed Kate grabbir handfuls of confetti and throwing them into the ai The girls kissed and hugged the happy coupl tears flowing and giggles erupting – Polly wa married, like a proper grown-up!

As the car drove off towards the airport, Chrissi turned back to the other three left behind. 'OK she said, 'let's go and get some big glasses c Champagne and toast the loss of another single gir They started off inside. 'Oh, not you, Laura,' sai Jaz, putting her hand to her mouth apologeticall 'You've got to go and see John, he's waiting for yo in the rose garden. I forgot to tell you, sorry.'

'Why?' asked Laura, nervously.

'I'm not sure,' cried Jaz over her shoulder. 'He ju said he had something to ask you ...'

index

13; ringlets 115, 118, 256, 285; rock chick 272–5; sexy plaits 113; short 'n' sweet 199; short and spiky 110; ki chic 187; spiky twists 137; stencilling 146; textured hair 94; top-knot scrunchies 137; twist and shout 200; twisted sister 70; uptown girl 144; va-va-voom 195; wavy hair 115; see also under wedding day
162, 170, 174, 180, 187
d massage 217
dbands 125
dscarves 65, 125, 165, 170, 174, 298
rt-shaped face 34, 170, 235
c-protection spray 161
lights see under colour
days: climate see climate; air enemies 164–5; hair prep 69–70; hair solutions 180; hair tips 174; quick fixes 211; tool kit 180, 187, 188, 192, 199, 200, 204

rview hair 66

ellery 125, 235, 262

atin 15, 162, 165

rs 34, 38, 66, 76, 134, 140, 169

on juice 225
tyle 15, 28, 75
face 34, 170
hair 38; curling tongs 89; utting 75, 76, 78–9; hidden colour 101; rock chick 110; uper-shiny 122; tied back 204, 11; updos 140; and wedding 244, 252, 262, 268, 272, 276, 80, 285, 298; and wigs 126; book' 42
lights see under colour

anin 162
length hair 169; 3-D lights 101; idden colour 101; at wedding 52, 262, 266, 268, 276, 280; erals 26, 221, 239
asse 23, 59, 92; 'bed-head' hair 5; colour 98, 170; holidays 92, 200, 204; 11; quick fixes 64; updos 66; olumizing 94; wedding day 291; iplait 113
ural drying 60
klaces 125, 144, 252, 262, 66, 276
tine 28
nal hair 16
ients 221, 239, 240, 240

hair see greasy/oily hair
face 34, 170
styling 246

panthenol (Provitamin B5) 23
parting 34, 36, 59, 76, 122, 123, 262
perfume 122, 174
piroctone olamine 19
plaits 98, 191, 268; decorating 113, 123, 256; fake 126; French 113, 142, 184; multiplait 113; sexy 113; unravelled 200, 252
pollution 19, 23, 28, 188
polymers 23
pomades 49, 65, 92, 98, 291
ponytails 66, 70, 192, 298; emergency quick fixes 128; extensions 122, 126; finger-combed 64; and hairpiece 144; high pony 134, 140, 207; holidays 180; tips 207

quick fixes 64, 128

ragging 115, 118
razor-cutting 126
red hair 170
restyles 36
reworkings 42
ribbons 146, 174, 180, 256, 266, 285
ringlets see under hairstyles
rock chick hair 76, 84, 94, 110, 272–5
rollers 89, 192, 294
roots: lift 60, 66, 89, 294; nourishment 15, 26
rough-drying 164
round face 34, 170

sand 165, 180
scalp: and brushes/combs 24; dry 16, 225; energizer 240; flaky 16, 26, 72, 225, 239, 246; greasy/oily 15, 16; massage 15, 26, 72, 217, 240; treatment 221, 225
scrumpling technique 276
sea salt 164, 180, 211, 217, 224, 225
seborrheic dermatitis 246
sebum 17, 24, 26; glands 16, 65, 225
sectioning clips 89
sequins 125
serum 23, 94; anti-frizz 92, 113, 162, 164, 199; basic blow-dry 58; and curls 17, 60, 256, 285; and fine hair 161, 162; and hair shaft 122, 161, 174; holidays 174, 204; and long hair 122; quick fixes 64, 128; and straight hair 17, 63; updos 66; wedding day 291
setting lotion 118, 134
setting spray 192
shading 49
shaggy style 110, 276
shampoos: baby 19; cheap 65; clarifying 224; for colour-treated hair 53, 170; dandruff 19, 225; deep-cleansing 221; designer 19;

detoxifying 19, 123, 174, 204, 217, 224; five-step shampoo 20; on holiday 161, 162, 174, 187, 188, 199, 200; moisturizing 162; pH-balanced 19; rehydrating 17
shine enhancer 92
shine spray 60, 113, 119, 195, 291, 294
short hair 38; 3-D lights 101; changing to 75, 76, 78–9; curling tongs 89; holidays 169, 211; quick fixes 64; styling options 110; and wax 298; and wedding 244, 245, 252, 256, 262, 266, 268, 276, 280, 298
silica 224
silicone 23, 65, 92, 92, 128
silver foil 118
skin tone 44, 98
SOS glamour kit 199
SOS tool kit 128
spiky hair 75, 110, 137, 262
split ends 15, 24, 38, 65, 162, 169, 217, 224, 225, 240
square face 34
static 23, 24, 27, 65, 72, 93, 161, 165
stencilling 146
straight hair 89; big 106; cold climate 161; condition of 17; creating ringlets 115, 118; and curls 76, 123, 245; 'Gucci-style' 110
straighteners 23, 64, 180, 244
straightening irons 63, 89
stress 15, 16, 26, 239
string, wet 66, 128, 134
styling: basic blow-dry 58; great curls 60; natural drying 60; quick fixes 64; secrets 94; straightening 63; style-and-go tips 65; tool kit 59
styling crème 92, 291
styling products: choosing 15, 23, 92–3; holidays 161, 165, 169, 174; overuse 298; wedding 240, 245, 291, 294
styling spray 59, 115, 128, 200
stylist's tool box 89
sun-protection products 17, 161, 162, 164, 165, 174, 180, 211
sunglasses 188, 211
supplements 15, 26, 27, 28, 239

tangles 24, 58, 59, 65, 89
textured hair 94, 101, 110, 262, 272, 276
texturizing 42, 94, 123; scissors 272
thickeners 93
thickening sprays 23
tiaras 125, 146, 235, 244, 246, 256, 266, 268, 272, 276, 280, 291, 294
tie-dying 56, 101
tocopherol 23

tonal blast 49, 101
tone on tone 49
top-knot scrunchies 137
towel-drying 164
travel plug 174
trichologist 246
twists 70, 146, 174, 192, 276; chopstick 207; spiky 137

ultraviolet (UV) light 28; and conditioners 164, 170, 174, 187, 188, 199, 200; free radicals 161; and keratin 162, 165; and melanin 162; oxidation 23; and shampoos 17, 170; sun-protection gel 211
updos 66, 83, 128, 291, 294; dos and don'ts 140; dressing 146; glam-hair 70; hairspray 93

vegetable colours 48, 98
vitamins 15, 20, 23, 26, 28, 221, 239
volume 42, 93, 192, 294; backcombing 146, 294; basic blow-dry 58; big hair 94, 192; and crimping 123; hairpieces 244; heated rollers 187; quick fixes 128; round brushes 89; straight hair 106; volumizing products 17, 23, 93, 264

washing hair 19–20, 53, 225
water: drinking 26, 72, 165, 174, 239; salt 164, 174
waves 76, 89, 115, 123, 164, 240, 280, 298
waving iron 252
waxes 23, 49, 92, 94, 98, 291, 298; 'bed-head' hair 65; choppy look 58; holidays 204; natural drying 60; and static 72; sun-protection 164
wedding day: Audrey style 264–5; beach style 284–5; boho vintage style 252–5; bridesmaids 240, 291; classic style 268–71; countdown 246; country style 256–9; fashionista style 276–7; finding a look 235; hair condition 239–40; hair products 291; making your hairstyle last 294; post-ceremony 298–9; pre-wedding hair tips 246; rock chick style 272–5; romantic style 280–83; SOS kit 294, 298; urbanite style 262–5; wedding wisdom 244–5
wedding dress 235, 244, 246, 252, 256, 266, 268, 276, 280, 285
wedding veils 235, 244, 246, 266, 268, 294
wheatgerm oil 20, 23
wigs 44, 75, 123, 126, 240
witch hazel 64

acknowledgements

Thank you to Adam Reed and Carolyn Newman
at the Percy Street salon.
With special thanks to Julie Gibson Jarvie, Penny Stock
and Venetia Penfold, without whom the book wouldn't
have been possible.

The publishers would like to thank the following for fashion loans for the shoot:
Lara Bohinc 107 (020 7405 7744), Elizabeth Emanuel (020 7486 7979),
Nicole Farhi (020 7499 8368), Joelynian (020 7267 4770),
Joseph (020 7225 3335) and Amanda Wakeley (020 7590 9105).

With special thanks to the following:

Bud (by appointment only), tel: 020 8537 0626

Butler & Wilson, 20 South Molton Street, London W1K 5QY, tel: 020 7409 2955

Isabel Kurtenbach Designs (by appointment only), tel: 020 7854 9647,
email: design@isabelkurtenbach.com, website:www.isabelkurtenbach.com

Nicola Pulvertaft (by appointment only), tel: 07747 792 082

Amanda Wakeley, 80 Fulham Road, London SW3 6HR, tel: 020 7590 9105

Basia Zarzycka (by appointment only), 52 Sloane Square, London SW1W 8AX, tel:
020 7730 1660, email: basia@basia.com, website: www.basias.com

2011   updated from our 2002 18y
10/12: 1x led 3/12   A 4
11/13: 4x led 5/13   A4 F4
12/14: 5y "   10/14
6/16:   7x "   6/16
10/8   9x "
8/19: 10x " 12/8